50 WAYS

to Prevent and Manage Stress

M. Sara Rosenthal

Contemporary Books

Chicago   New York   San Francisco   Lisbon   London   Madrid   Mexico City
Milan   New Delhi   San Juan   Seoul   Singapore   Sydney   Toronto

Library of Congress Cataloging-in-Publication Data

Rosenthal, M. Sara.
    50 ways to prevent and manage stress / M. Sara Rosenthal.
      p.   cm.
    Includes bibliographical references and index.
    ISBN 0-7373-0558-4 (alk. paper)
    1. Stress (Psychology).   2. Stress management.   I. Title: Fifty ways to prevent and
manage stress.   II. Title.

BF575.S75 R66   2001
155.9'042—dc21   2001028879

Contemporary Books

A Division of The McGraw-Hill Companies

1 2 3 4 5 6 7 8 9 0   DOC/DOC   0 9 8 7 6 5 4 3 2 1

ISBN 0-7373-0558-4

This book was set in Cochin
Printed and bound by R. R. Donnelley

McGraw-Hill books are available at special quantity discounts to use as premiums and sales promotions, or
for use in corporate training programs. For more information, please write to the Director of Special Sales,
Professional Publishing, McGraw-Hill, Two Penn Plaza, New York, NY 10121-2298. Or contact your local
bookstore.

The purpose of this book is to educate. It is sold with the understanding that the author and publisher shall
have neither liability nor responsibility for any injury caused or alleged to be caused directly or indirectly by
the information contained in this book. While every effort has been made to ensure the book's accuracy, its
contents should not be construed as medical advice. Each person's health needs are unique. To obtain
recommendations appropriate to your particular situation, please consult a qualified health care provider.

This book is printed on acid-free paper.

Contents

Acknowledgments

I wish to thank the following people, whose expertise on past works helped to lay so much of the groundwork for this book: Gillian Arsenault, M.D., C.C.F.P., I.B.L.C., F.R.C.P.; Pamela Craig, M.D., F.A.C.S., Ph.D.; Masood Kahthamee, M.D., F.A.C.O.G.; Debra Lander, M.D., F.R.C.P.C.; Mark Lander, M.D., F.R.C.P.C.; Sheila Lander, L.P.N./R.N.; Gary May, M.D., F.R.C.P.; James McSherry, M.B., Ch.B., F.C.F.P., F.R.C.G.P., F.A.A.F.P., F.A.B.M.P.; Suzanne Pratt, M.D., F.A.C.O.G.; Wm. Warren H. Rudd, M.D., F.R.C.S.(C.), F.A.C.S., Fellow, A.S.C.R.S.; and Robert Volpe, M.D., F.R.C.P., F.A.C.P. Larissa Kostoff, my editorial consultant, worked very hard to help bring this book into being. Finally, Hudson Perigo, my editor, offered many wonderful and thoughtful suggestions to help make this book what it is.

Other books by M. Sara Rosenthal:

The Thyroid Sourcebook

The Gynecological Sourcebook

The Pregnancy Sourcebook

The Fertility Sourcebook

The Breastfeeding Sourcebook

The Breast Sourcebook

The Gastrointestinal Sourcebook

Managing Your Diabetes *

Managing Diabetes for Women *

The Type 2 Diabetic Woman

The Thyroid Sourcebook for Women

Women and Sadness *

Women and Depression

Women of the '60s Turning 50 *

Women and Passion *

50 Ways to Prevent Colon Cancer

50 Ways Women Can Prevent Heart Disease

50 Ways to Manage Heartburn, Reflux, and Ulcers

50 Ways to Manage Type 2 Diabetes

50 Ways to Prevent Depression

SarahealthGuides® (These are M. Sara Rosenthal's own line of health books dedicated to rare, controversial, or stigmatizing health topics; they are available only at online bookstores such as amazon.com.):

Stopping Cancer at the Source

Women and Unwanted Hair

---

*(in Canada only or online through www.chapters.ca)

Introduction

What Is Stress?

Generally, stress is a negative emotional experience associated with biological changes that trigger your body to make adaptations. For example, in response to stress, your adrenal glands pump out *stress hormones* that speed up your body. Your heart rate increases, and your blood sugar levels rise so that your body can divert glucose to your muscles in case you have to flee dangerous situations. Together, these changes are known as the *fight or flight response*. The stress hormones, technically called the *catecholamines*, are broken down into epinephrine (adrenaline) and norepinephrine.

The problem with stress hormones in the twenty-first century is that the fight or flight response is rarely necessary. Today most stress stems from interpersonal situations rather than from attacks by a predator. Occasionally, you may want to flee from a bank robber or mugger, but most of us just want to flee from our jobs or our kids! As a result, your stress hormones actually put a physical strain on your body and can lower your resistance to disease. Initially, stress hormones stimulate your immune system, but after the stressful event has passed, they can suppress the immune system, leaving you open to a wide variety of illnesses and physical symptoms.

Hans Selye, considered the father of stress management, defined stress as the wear and tear on the body. Once you are in a state of stress, the body adapts to the stress by depleting its resources until it becomes exhausted. The wear and tear on your body is mounting; you can suffer from stress-related conditions:

- Allergies and asthma
- Back pain
- Cardiovascular problems
- Dental and periodontal problems
- Depression
- Emotional outbursts (rage, anger, crying, irritation—seen in recent reports on "air rage" and "desk rage")
- Fatigue
- Gastrointestinal problems (digestive disorders, bowel problems, and so on)
- Headaches
- Herpes recurrences (especially in women)
- High blood pressure
- High cholesterol
- Immune suppression (predisposing us to viruses, such as colds and flu, infections, autoimmune disorders, and cancer)

- Insomnia
- Loss of appetite and weight loss
- Muscular aches and pains
- Premature aging
- Sexual problems
- Skin problems and rashes

As you can see from this lengthy list, stress greatly contributes to ill health and disease. Addictions and substance abuse may fuel many of these problems when you try to relieve your symptoms or self-medicate. Current statistics reveal that 43 percent of all adults suffer from health problems directly caused by stress, while 70 to 90 percent of all visits to primary-care physicians are for stress-related complaints or disorders. In the workplace alone, about a million people per day call in sick because of stress. That rate translates into about 550 million absences per year. Other studies show that roughly 50 percent of all North American workers suffer from *burnout*—a state of mental exhaustion and fatigue caused by stress—and that 40 percent of employee turnover is directly caused by stress.

The financial toll of occupational stress on North American industry adds up to about $300 billion annually. This figure includes costs of absenteeism, lower productivity, employee turnover, and direct medical, legal, and insurance fees. California employers alone spend about $1 billion for medical and legal fees due to stress. Ninety percent of job stress lawsuits are successful, and the resulting fines are four times those for other injury claims. Meanwhile, corporate spending on stress management programs grew from $9.4 billion in 1995 to $11.3 billion in 1999.

The consequences of stress can be worse than these financial ones. Terrible industry accidents such as oil spills or nuclear reactor accidents are considered to be caused— 60 to 80 percent of the time—by overstressed workers. Terms such as *office rage* and *desk rage* are emerging, too, as workplace violence escalates. A more subtle but compelling statistic is this: In 1997, the Japanese word *karoshi*, which means sudden death from overwork, began appearing in English dictionaries.

Types of Stress

Managing your stress is no easy feat, particularly since there are different types of stress: acute stress and chronic stress. Acute stress results from an acute situation, such as a sudden, unexpected negative event or a difficult task like organizing a wedding or planning for a conference. When the event passes or the task ends, the stress goes away. Acute stress has numerous symptoms: anger or irritability, anxiety, depression, tension headaches or migraines, back pain, jaw pain, muscular tension, digestive problems, cardiovascular problems, and dizziness.

Acute stress can be *episodic*, meaning that one stressful event follows another, creating a continuous flow of acute stress. Someone who is always taking on too many projects at once may suffer from episodic acute stress, rather than simply acute stress. Workaholics and those with the so-called *Type A* personality (i.e., perfectionists) are classic sufferers of episodic acute stress.

I sometimes refer to acute stress as the *good stress*. Often, good things come from this kind of stress, even though it feels stressful or bad in the short term. Acute stress challenges us to stretch ourselves beyond our capabilities. It is what makes us meet deadlines, push the outside of the envelope, and invent creative solutions to our problems. Consider a few examples of good stress:

- Challenging projects
- Positive life-changing events (moving, changing jobs, or ending unhealthy relationships)
- Confronting fears, illnesses, or people that make us feel bad

These situations can be difficult to endure, but often the outcome is good for us in the long term.

Essentially, whenever a stressful event triggers emotional, intellectual, or spiritual growth, it is a good stress. It is often not the event itself but your *response* to the event that determines whether it is a good or bad stress. Even the death of a loved one can sometimes lead to personal growth. For example, we may see something about ourselves we did not see before, such as new resilience. In this case, grieving a death can be a good stress, though we are sad in the short term.

What I call the *bad stress* is known as chronic stress. Chronic stress results from boredom and stagnation, as well as prolonged negative circumstances. Essentially, when no growth occurs from the stressful event, it is bad stress. When negative events don't seem to yield anything positive in the long term, but more of the same, the stress can lead to chronic and debilitating health problems. Some examples of bad stress include stagnant jobs or relationships, disability from terrible accidents or diseases, long-term unemployment, chronic poverty, racism, or lack of opportunities for change. These kinds of situations can lead to depression, low self-esteem, and a host of physical illnesses.

In addition to acute and chronic stress, stress can be defined in even more precise ways:

- Physical stress (from physical exertion)
- Chemical stress (from exposure to a toxin in the environment, including from substance abuse)
- Mental stress (from taking on too much responsibility and worrying about all that has to be done)
- Emotional stress (from feelings such as anger, fear, frustration, sadness, betrayal, or bereavement)
- Nutritional stress (from deficiency in certain vitamins or nutrients, overindulgence in fat or protein, or food allergies)
- Traumatic stress (from trauma to the body such as infection, injury, burns, surgery, or extreme temperatures)
- Psychospiritual stress (from unrest in your personal relationships or belief system, personal life goals, and so on—in general, the factors that define whether or not you are happy)

The bottom line is that *stress can make you sick*. This book is designed to help you reorganize your priorities so that you can reduce chronic stress as well as incorporate a few new healing strategies to help combat acute stress. Finding ways to downshift (Items 1 through 10) while incorporating hands-on healing (Items 11 through 20), herbs and nutrients (Items 21 through 30), inner and outer workouts (Items 31 through 40), and self-care (Items 41 through 50) into your daily routine may dramatically reduce your current stresses.

PART ONE

Downshifting

1. Recognize How Hard You Work

Downshifting is a term that emerged in the early 1990s to mean *slowing down*. The first step in downshifting is to recognize the *need* to do so. You may not be aware of how much stress you endure by simply working in the nine-to-five workplace (which is more like five to nine for many) that still exists in most offices. The workplace is a volatile *stress factory* for most employees. One reason is the constant threat of losing your job, as mergers and downsizing have increased job stress for millions. Another source of stress is the unspoken pressure to put in *face time,* or hang around the office longer to look like you're productive and dedicated, even though no one has directly told you to stay. Factor in new bosses, computer surveillance, and fewer health and retirement benefits, and it's easy to see how workplace stress can affect your personal life.

One of the most significant factors in job stress is a sense of powerlessness over your job or duties. Secretaries, waitresses, middle managers, police officers, editors, and medical interns are considered high-stress positions because these jobs entail a lot of responsibility but little authority. Another stressful mismatch is to be a poet in a desk job— that is, to be a highly creative person performing an unchallenging job to pay the rent. For example, are you an actor by night and a bookkeeper or receptionist by day?

A number of studies note that when you don't control decision making in your workplace, you endure more chronic stress. Although acute stress often comes with the responsibility of making decisions, people are more motivated and challenged creatively when they feel their opinions or decisions are valued.

Jobs also may cause trauma. Criminal justice personnel, firefighters, ambulance drivers, military personnel, and disaster teams witness horrific scenes each day. Physicians, caregivers, social workers, and therapists experience vicarious traumatization, meaning that they are traumatized by what they see and hear through their clients each day. Even ordinary jobs can be traumatic when clients emotionally or physically threaten you.

The workplace itself can be stressful to your physique if it is hazardous or toxic in some way. In 1995, Dr. Peter Inante, Director of the Office of Standards Review, Occupational Safety and Health Administration of the U.S. Department of Labor, stated that blue-collar workers "appeared to be the canaries in our society for identifying human chemical carcinogens in the general environment." Known carcinogens at the office (or home) may be found in many places:

- Asbestos building materials
- Cleaning products and disinfectants

- Urea-formaldehyde foam insulation
- Adhesives (may contain naphthalene, phenol, ethanol, vinyl chloride, formaldehyde, acrylonitrile, and epoxy, which are toxic substances that release vapors)
- Toners used in copy machines and printers
- Particleboard furniture and space dividers
- Permanent-ink pens and markers (contain acetone, cresol, ethanol, phenol, toluene, and xylene)
- Polystyrene cups
- Secondhand smoke
- Synthetic office carpet (may contain acrylic, polyester, and nylon plastic fibers and formaldehyde-based finishes) or wool carpet (may contain pesticides for mothproofing)
- Correction fluid, such as Wite-Out or Liquid Paper brands (may contain cresol, ethanol, trichloroethylene, and naphthalene, which are all toxic chemicals)

You're more likely to be affected by workplace carcinogens if you are subject to one or more of the following conditions:

- Work or live in energy-sealed buildings
- Are exposed to fumes from carpets, pesticides, cleaners, and airborne allergens
- Are exposed to industrial chemicals, such as those found in plants that process wood, metal, plastics, paints, and textiles

- Are in constant contact with pesticides, fungicides, and fertilizers
- Live in high-pollution areas
- Work in dry cleaning, hair styling, pest control, printing, or photocopying

For more information, you can go to the NIOSH-TIC database, maintained by the National Institute for Occupational Safety and Health (NIOSH) and available on the Internet. You can also call NIOSH Information Dissemination at (513) 533-8287. Other government agencies with relevant information are the Centers for Disease Control and Prevention (CDC) in Atlanta, Georgia — (404) 639-3311 — and the Occupational Safety and Health Administration (OSHA), which is the federal agency in charge of workplace safety and health.

2. At Least *Try* to Do What You Love

If you do what you love, you'll love what you do. And you'll feel so much better, even though you may not make as much money. Surveys and studies show across the board that daily going to a job you hate creates stress.

Doing what you love doesn't necessarily mean throwing in the towel and moving to France so you can paint for the rest of your life. It means exploring what you're good at (and/or enjoy doing) to see if there's a way you can earn an income from it. For example, can you take courses that would allow you to enter a field you prefer? The promise of a more satisfying future achieved with the right credentials often reduces chronic stress arising from the prospect of the same old same old. Although expanding your education or training may involve some short-term stress from the added responsibilities, in the long term it gives you a more hopeful future, which in turn will reduce stress.

Sometimes doing what you love means accepting that you're not very good at management and would prefer a nonmanagerial position. For many people, the solution is to work in the store instead of running it. On the flip side, you may find that doing what you love means facing the fact that you *are* a leader and find it stressful to be in a subordinate position. In this case, perhaps starting your own company (where you have control) may be less stressful, even though it involves far more responsibility. Although many have failed, there are still some who have found success starting Internet businesses and home-based businesses, taking advantage of new technologies and access to a global market through the Internet. Another way to satisfy a craving for control or leadership is to move to positions in large companies that allow you to start a new venture as an "intrapreneur," or a manager with an entrepreneur's authority. Millions of other independent-minded employees work as traveling salespeople, who receive a gas or car allowance and work mostly on commission with a small base salary. These positions offer the flexibility and the control of lifestyle that can enable employees to feel autonomous.

Some people can't support themselves by doing what they love, so they downshift by moving to a simple side job with flexible hours. The side job pays the bills, and the flexible schedule allows time for art or another main interest. Couriers, postal workers, restaurant servers, and so forth frequently have more artistic lifestyles. If a job simply supports your art, it is less important than a job that is part of your career. A side job is less stressful because it doesn't consume your life. If you lose one side job, it's easy to get another. In other words, side jobs involve *detachment*, while career-jobs involve attachment and far more emotional investment. Sometimes doing what you love means facing up to the fact that your dream job or profession has become a living nightmare. This is not an easy thing to admit, because it often demands a major change. For example, imagine an overworked medical resident in a busy university teaching hospital. When she admits she spends most of her time filling out insurance paperwork, she decides that she's packing up and becoming a country doctor in an underserviced rural area. She won't become the brilliant heart surgeon her family dreamed of; she won't earn $350,000 per year, not including the conference perks. Instead, she'll settle for a third of that salary in a rural setting where the housing is affordable and people say hello to her.

Pursuing what you love involves four steps:

1. Ask yourself whether you're happy with your choice of job or career. Being happy is not the same thing as feeling *stable* or *not miserable*. If you're not happy, persisting in a state of unhappiness is unhealthy.

2. Make a list of dream jobs or careers, no matter how silly you think you're being. Always wanted to be a dancer, but are making a living in marketing? Maybe you can pursue administrative or marketing jobs with a dance company or dance theater. Maybe you can write about dance or start a children's dance school. Always wanted to be a farmer? Why not? Organic farming is booming! Dream jobs can also mean parenting. If being a stay-at-home parent is your dream, it's worth pursuing, too.

3. Assess whether you hate your profession, or just your job or locale. How portable is your profession? If you have a job that's in demand everywhere, like Webmaster, writer, or teacher, find a more suitable city or town to live in, and just start working. The Internet can make many careers portable. Are you a burned-out secretary? Start your own secretarial services company on the Web. (If there isn't a "secretary.com" yet, someone should start one!)

4. Talk to your family members, and seek their support to pursue something else. If your family members are not behind you, pursuing what you love may be more difficult and may make you face deep questions about your emotional support system. Pursuing your dreams sometimes requires leaving relationships or marriage. In assessing what you want, you may discover that all these years, you've been living behind a mask or simply going through the motions of your existence.

3. Reduce the Commute

One of the simplest ways to destress and downshift is to eliminate that stressful commute. If you live in a bedroom community and drive into an urban center, you may be spending more than an hour each way, to and from work. Driving is stressful, and reducing the drive can reduce a lot of stress. Here are some ways to reduce your commute:

- If you spend most of your time at work on the computer or on the phone, try to negotiate telecommuting with your employer. This means being plugged into the office from home. With teleconferencing tools, there's little reason to actually go into an office these days. Your employer can save on overhead because of the office space you'll free up, and the flexibility may attract more loyal employees.

- Look into moving closer to work. If you calculate your car expenses, gas expenses, and so on, moving within walking distance to work may be the answer. Many people find trading a house in the suburbs for a rental in the city makes more sense financially. Rent and no car often equal far less than a mortgage and two cars! Car rentals for weekends away and the occasional taxi still add up to less than car lease payments, car financing payments, car repairs, gas, maintenance, and insurance.

- If there's no way you can move, no way your employer will let you work from home, and you're working very late hours anyway, consider renting a small apartment or room within walking distance of your office. Leave the car at the office weekdays, and crash in your small city space. Drive home for the weekends. Of course, if this creates more stress, don't do it, but a lot of commuters are finding a small city crash pad has other advantages. You can extend the "pad" to visiting friends or relatives (often hosting visitors creates more stress!), and other family members can use the pad when they have to be in the city for extended periods of time. Sometimes marriages and long-term relationships benefit when there's a place to go for personal space or distance in high-stress times.

4. Reduce Your Workweek

Moving down from a five-day workweek to a four-day workweek greatly reduces stress for many. Psychologically, working Tuesday to Friday eliminates Mondays. According to Deepak Chopra, more people have heart attacks Monday mornings than any other time. Another popular choice is to work Monday to Thursday, giving you an early start to your weekend. If you're a valued employee, many employers would rather have you working four days for them than not at all. When you calculate the time it takes to train someone else, it's more costly to replace you than to give you a four-day week. You simply reduce your salary to accommodate your new workweek.

Another way to negotiate a reduced workweek is to use vacation and sick days as *Mondays off* for a year. Some executives have accumulated weeks of unused vacation time, which they can use for reduced workweeks. In some companies, being away from the office for long periods of time actually creates more stress and guilt for the employee. Taking a day off each week may be one solution to "vacationitis."

You might also be able to reduce your workweek by finding someone else at work who wants to share a job. Surveys show that most people would trade full-time hours for part-time hours if they could have job security.

5. Renegotiate Vacation and Leave Time

In a study of 12,338 men ages thirty-five to fifty-seven, the American Psychosomatic Society found that men who took annual vacations were 21 percent less likely to die during the sixteen-year study period than were nonvacationers —

and 32 percent less likely to die of coronary heart disease. This is not at all surprising. Two weeks of vacation time is not enough for the average person. European companies routinely offer six weeks of vacation. When you renegotiate your vacation package, offer to combine paid vacation with unpaid leave. Surveys show that most people would gladly take unpaid vacation time if they were guaranteed job security.

A more dramatic move is to look into taking sabbatical leave. This means taking a year off for *family reasons* (stress reduction, mental health, etc.) without pay, and returning to work the next year. Many people would take a year off if they could be guaranteed job security upon returning. Sabbatical leave is offered to some professionals, such as teachers and tenured professors at universities, but there's no reason why it should not be an option for other professions. Cashing in some retirement funds to finance your sabbatical year could pay off in the form of rejuvenation.

6. Rid Yourself of E-Stress

For most people, E-mail, voice mail, cellular phones, fax machines, pagers, and the host of technology that is part of our lives have only lengthened our workdays and given us less time to ourselves. The greater access to communication that technology provides makes our "To Do" lists much longer. Twenty-five years ago, when you called someone who wasn't home, the phone rang many times, and that was it. There was not an onus on the person called to return your call; the onus was on the caller to try again. But with voice mail, the onus is on the called to return the call—or with the advent of call waiting, to answer numerous calls simultaneously. Today, avoiding phone calls requires even more technology, lest we appear to be antisocial by screening our calls.

And if you've made the mistake of subscribing to list servers, you could become bombarded with E-mail — as many as hundreds of messages per day. The benefits and burden of technology increase with handheld organizers, laptop computers, and so forth. Even watching television has become infinitely more complicated, with complex remotes that not only power the VCR and stereo system but also can rewire your house!

All this translates into the term *E-stress*. Part of E-stress is the learning curve. Learning each new technology toy can wreak havoc on the central nervous system of many. And the learning, it seems, never ends, as new gadgets keep being introduced and making the old gadgets obsolete. New versions of E-mail software or fax software also are problematic.

Another part of E-stress is lack of privacy. With so many ways to be contacted, there is no safe haven that is communication-free. In addition, overly loud cell-phone conversations force us to listen to someone else's private life in public places. We've all had those moments where we've glared at someone because we really didn't need to know about her mother's friend's colonoscopy! With each new mode of communication come new responsibilities to reply. Experts call this situation *multitasking madness*.

All the "E" in your life interferes with normal communication. When you're E-mailing with one hand, talking on the phone with the other, and feeling your pager go off in the same instant, how much focused communication can you deliver or receive? The first step in turning down the "E" is looking at all the ways you're plugged in each day. Ask yourself these questions:

- How many phone lines do you have?

- How do you receive the Internet? If it's via cable or dedicated line, you're never off.

- How many ways can people reach you?

- How many messages do you receive through each mode of communication? Count everything: E-mail to your office, E-mail to your home, phone messages to your cell phone, your office phone, your voice mail, and so on.

- Does E-mail enhance your interpersonal relationships or detract from them? For example, do you find yourself feeling isolated in spite of all the ways you can contact people? Does your life partner spend time with you at home—or with his or her computer? Do your children spend quality time at home, or do they spend all of their time on-line or playing video and computer games? A 2000 Stanford University study on the societal impact of the Internet found that Internet use caused social isolation, which supported the findings of a 1998 study by researchers at Carnegie Mellon University.

The preceding questions are designed to help you evaluate the impact of the "E" in your life. Reducing E-stress involves redesigning the technology in your life to work *for* you rather than against you. By implementing just one of these steps, you can help reduce E-stress:

- Set up unplugged time. Make a decision to be unplugged by a certain time of day, such as after

6:00 P.M. and on weekends. You can even indicate your unplug zone on your outgoing voice mail: "Hi. You've reached Dale at 555-5555. I check my voice mail between nine and six each day. After that time, I cannot be reached." Turn off your computer after 6:00 P.M., too, and do not check E-mail beyond a certain time. You can also set up automatic E-mail responses that tell people you're away, busy, not answering, and so on.

- Use your cell phone only in case of emergency: for outgoing emergency calls only in case of accident or something unexpected. Don't give out the number to anyone other than very close family members, and don't turn it on except in an emergency. If you have voice mail and E-mail, people don't really need to reach you by cell phone. Don't subscribe to a message service on your cell phone, either. That way, no one *can* leave messages.

- Limit your gadgets. If you've survived this long without a Palm device, do you *really* need one? In other words, the more stuff you buy, the more you'll use, and the less time you'll have.

- Limit your surfing time. If you're searching for information about a topic on the Internet (such as stress!), you can be there for days. Give yourself a limited amount of time for research, and then say (as I do), "I've done the best I can with the time I have."

- Limit the messages you save. Try to write down the information as you get it, and erase the messages. Otherwise, you'll spend too much time listening to old messages.

- Eliminate phone tag by leaving a specific message with specific instructions for replying: "Hi, George, this is Su Lin. I wanted to set up a meeting this Thursday, at 1:00 P.M., in front of the Coffee Mill. If you can't make it, E-mail me with an alternate time and place. Otherwise, I'll see you Thursday."

7. Eliminate Energy Drains

Most energy drains come in the form of people. When you're surrounded by people who take energy from you, rather than give you energy in the form of support, the result is more stress in your life. By seriously reevaluating your personal relationships, you may be able to find more energy and reduce the amount of stress in your life. Ask yourself the following questions:

- Does someone in your life offer judgment-free emotional support? This means a person who makes you feel positive about yourself rather than a person who points out your flaws or attacks your choices.

- Do some people in your life drain your energy and reserves? These are people who always seem to be in crisis and suck up large amounts of "free therapy" time from you but never seem to be there for you. These can also be people who criticize you and make you feel negative and hopeless instead of positive and optimistic.

- Do you have unresolved conflicts with family members or friends? These unresolved feelings can drain your energy and focus, as we tend to obsess over the conflict (see Item 50).

- Do you feel your friends are really only acquaintances? Do you lack truly intimate friendships?

- Do you feel a void in your life because there is an absence of a romantic partner?

- Are you in a romantic or sexual relationship that you need to end, but you have been avoiding action?

- Are you in a relationship that compromises your values?

- Is there a phone call you need to make, but are avoiding, that is causing you stress and anxiety?

- Does someone in your life continuously break commitments or plans, so you are constantly rescheduling?

Energy drains can also come from unmet needs in your home environment. Do you have broken appliances, a car in need of repairs, a wardrobe you hate, cluttered closets and rooms, or even ugly surroundings? Living in a home that is not decorated in a way that pleases you makes you feel as though you don't want to be there. Plants, fresh paint, covers for ugly furniture, and a few beautiful prints or posters on the wall often make the difference between barren and cozy surroundings. See the section on Self-Care for more on the little things in life that make huge differences in your stress quotient.

Other energy drains come from procrastinating and over-booking yourself. We will procrastinate over things we really don't want to do—such as paying taxes. We overbook ourselves when we're afraid of saying no. Every article and book on stress management has these three trite words of advice: Just say no. The problem is, few people will ever say that. Instead of "No," try, "Let me check my schedule and see if I'm already committed." Then you can say, "Sorry, it looks like I'm committed elsewhere," or if the request is for you to complete a task, "I've got a deadline on that date for something equally important."

Finally, simply doing too much and expecting too much from ourselves drains our energies. When possible, hire someone to do the things you can't or don't want to do.

When you're overworked at the office, your employer may allow you to subcontract one or two projects to a freelancer. If you don't think your employer will pay for the freelancer, have you considered subbing out the dreaded task on the sly and paying for it out of your own pocket? The job security, perceived good performance, and weight off your shoulders may be worth a couple of hundred bucks. The same principle applies at home. Consider hiring someone to do these chores that many people dread:

- Cleaning your house or apartment
- Decluttering your house by going through closets, filing papers, and so on
- Organizing your tax receipts
- Gardening or taking care of your lawn

8. Reduce Your Snail Mail and Plastic

Mail is stressful. Do you have what I call that "dining room table problem"? Does your mail get sorted and piled on the dining room table night after night, to the point where the surface of the table disappears and you can never have company, because that would mean sorting your mail? If so, you probably have unnecessary mail. Calling companies and requesting that your name be removed from mailing lists is often just *another* thing we have do, so it doesn't get done.

The easiest way to reduce the mail that comes inside your door is to place a garbage can or recycling bin right by your mailbox so you can sort the mail outside the door. All flyers and direct mailings (people asking for donations or selling new products, credit cards, or services) go immediately into the garbage. Don't even open them! Postcards, thank-you notes, and so on should get read on the spot, but unless you feel some dire need to save them, toss them out, too.

The next task is going through your bills and figuring out what can get paid by phone or on-line. Can you request a stop on snail-mail bills and ask for E-mail billings? Can you prepay or arrange to have bills automatically paid by credit card or debit card and just get notice of monthly payments (such as utilities) on your credit card bill?

As for the plastic, so much mail and stress are generated by credit cards that it's amazing. If you have too many credit cards, you're probably spending more than you can afford and accumulating massive debts. The best credit cards to have are cards that give you something in return, such as frequent-flier miles. Pick one card, and *fly* with it! Or pick two—one for personal use and one for business use. Toss all the department store cards (and the various loyalty programs attached to them, which can mean more cards). Whenever someone calls to ask if I'm a member of some club that gives me something useless for free when I spend five hundred dollars at one store, I just say, "No, thanks."

Before you cut up the cards you're not using, be sure to pay the account in full. Also, tell the credit card company you're closing your account.

Finally, try to reduce your newspaper and magazine clutter by getting a few of them on-line. Most daily papers are now on-line, for example. At the very least, you can get the local information you need in the on-line edition.

9. Restructure Your Finances

Debt is stressful. Feeling the pressures of saving for retirement also can be stressful. While reducing your plastic is one small way of restructuring your finances, you can also restructure finances by *restructuring your life* so you're financing as little as possible. Here are some ways to do that:

- Get rid of your mortgage. If your house is mortgaged to the hilt or in need of expensive renovations that you can't afford, that's stressful. Many people find that selling the "money pit" house and buying or renting something cheaper eliminates a lot of debt and stress.

- Get rid of your car. If you're a two-car family, try living with only one car. If you're a one-car family, getting rid of a car is usually possible only in large urban centers with good public transit. Try living car-free for a year, and see if it makes a difference financially. Gas, repairs, insurance, tickets, parking, and car payments really add up.

- Use retirement funds to pay off credit card debts or other nagging debts. Your retirement savings don't have to be used just for retirement. You're saving your money to help yourself in the future. Maybe the time to use some of that money is now. Get rid of those high-interest debts once and for all. Perhaps the money you save by not paying interest can go back into your savings account. Consult a financial adviser before deciding which strategy would be best for you.

- **Resist the pressure to play the market.** There is a lot of pressure from fund management companies to invest your money in high-risk stocks or money-market accounts in exchange for higher interest. You could certainly make money on these ventures—but you can lose your money, too. If you can't afford to lose, you may not want to play. Keeping your money in guaranteed-interest accounts or lower-interest accounts that are less volatile may give you peace of mind—something perhaps more valuable than a piece of the action! When you consider the time spent on checking the stock market, worrying about the stock market, and so on, it's a lot of wasted energy. Getting your time back from the stock market may be more valuable than the stock itself.

10. Stop the Insanity: Stress Relief for Parents

One of the chief causes of stress for many is what's involved these days in raising kids. The onslaught of media and advertisements from all sides is creating in parents a perception that they need to give their children more stuff than the children actually need or want. In suburban or affluent communities, the amount of activities and money invested in children is staggering. And a lot of it is unnecessary. Children need love, roots, and wings. They don't need to be booked up twenty-four/seven with "play dates," various lessons, and an endless string of lavish birthday parties hosted by parents trying to outdo one another in themes, gifts, or entertainment. The more stuff you involve your children in, the more running around you have to do, and the more stressed and tired the child gets (not to mention you!). In the end, you have less time to spend with your children. Here are a few tips I've mined from parents who have downshifted their children:

Limit the Lessons

Your child does not need to be occupied with a different sport or art form every night of the week. If you want to expose the child to variety, try one different thing each school term until something sticks. One team sport or activity during the week is just fine. This will greatly reduce the amount of running around your family does, and the change will pay off in more quality family time.

Stop the Birthday Insanity

Some of these birthday survival tips are more doable or practical for some parents than others. But take a look:

- When your child reaches an age of understanding, consider the gift of charity for the next birthday party he or she attends. Donate an affordable amount (say, ten dollars) to a children's charity in the name of the birthday child. That's your gift. No more last-minute gift-shopping madness for a kid you don't know, who already has everything! When it's your turn to host a birthday party, request *no gifts*, but donations to your child's charity of choice are welcome. This will reduce the toy clutter, the greed factor, and the inequality factor (when some children give lavish presents and other children give cheaper presents, social dynamics can become nightmarish all around). Reserve gift giving for the family party you have for your child, and impress upon your child that the kids' party is designed for enjoying friends, not collecting material possessions.

- Limit the party's size. Most parents agree, "Eight is enough." Eight children or fewer is a manageable size. By limiting the amount of guests, you can limit your costs and the number of gifts your child receives. Entertain 1970s style with hot dogs or pizza, a cake, and some creative party games. Don't feel pressured to take the kids on a lavish outing.

- Reduce and reuse party gifts. Allow your child to choose a few gifts to keep and a few gifts to donate. You can use gifts from the "donate" pile for other parties, or give them all away to children's charities.

Living Child-Free

If you're delaying having children until your career is more settled or you feel more financially secure, have you considered the option of *not* having a child at all? In the past, a child-free lifestyle was a political decision for many couples. During the 1950s and 1960s, many couples chose this because they feared a nuclear holocaust. By the 1970s, the issue of overpopulation became the motivating factor for the choice. Yet by the 1980s, the option became unpopular. This is a pity, considering what a liberating lifestyle option it can be. Obviously, you'll need to review your original reasons for wanting children before you make this choice. You might want talk to child-free people to see if they regret the choice.

Having and raising children are one of the most stressful experiences in life. As an author of many women's health books, I can tell you that several women have said to me, "If I knew how hard raising children would be, I wouldn't have chosen it." Parenting is a selfless, largely self-sacrificing job. Choosing a child-free lifestyle may be an appealing option in an economically turbulent and difficult world.

Some of the traditional reasons for having children were purely economic. Children, many people thought, guaranteed financial security in old age. Today, with so many college-educated adults living at home because they cannot get jobs, the economic benefits of progeny are no longer as visible.

Another traditional reason for having children was fear of loneliness in one's old age. Fifteen years from now, the majority of the population will be over sixty-five; you won't be lonely.

Child-free living offers the following benefits:

- *Freedom.* You may have the time and extra money down the road to do all the things you've dreamed of: going back to school for that second degree, buying a vacation home, traveling, taking early retirement, or whatever you want.

- *Control of your life.* When you have children, you lose a certain control over your own life, as you become entangled in the precarious nature of parenting a child who lives on planet Earth. Children can have lots of problems: they may have difficulty at school, get sick, have accidents, get in trouble, and so on. Being a parent never stops.

- *Self-expansion.* You'll have the time to explore parts of yourself that you never knew existed, because you'll have time to yourself. You can explore insights about your life, your gifts, your talents, your desires, and your interests.

PART TWO

Hands-On Healing

11. Discover Your Life-Force Energy

Many ancient, non-Western cultures, be they in native North America, India, China, Japan, or ancient Greece, believed that there are two fundamental aspects to the human body. There is the actual physical shell (clinically called the corporeal body), consisting of cells, blood, tissue, and so on. In addition, they believed there is an energy flow that makes the physical body come alive. This energy flow was known as the *life force* or *life energy*.

In fact, the life force was so central to the view of human function that each non-Western culture has a word for it. In China it is called *qi* (pronounced "chee"). In India it's called *prana*, and in Japan it's called *ki*. The ancient Greeks called it *pneuma*, which has become a prefix in medical terms referring to breath and lungs.

Today, Western medicine concentrates on the corporeal body and does not recognize that we have a life force. However, non-Western, ancient healing presumes that the life force heals the corporeal body.

Every non-Western healer looks upon the parts of the body as *windows* or *maps* to the body's health. In Chinese medicine, the ears are a complex map, with each point on the ear representing a different organ or part of the psyche. In reflexology (discussed in Item 15), the map is the feet, which can tell a reflexologist much about the rest of the body and spirit. In Ayurvedic medicine, the tongue is read, while other traditions read the iris of the eyes or other parts of the body.

Western medicine doesn't really do this. Instead, it looks at every individual part for symptoms of a disease and treats each part individually. So, let's say you notice blurred vision. You might go to an eye doctor, who gives you a prescription for glasses and sends you on your way. But if you were to go to a Chinese medicine doctor, the doctor might tell you that the degeneration of your eyes points to an unhealthy liver. To the Chinese, the eyes are a direct window into the liver. (Interestingly, it is the eyes that turn yellow when you're jaundiced.) Instead of writing a simple prescription for glasses, the Chinese healer will look into deeper causes of this liver imbalance in the body. The doctor will ask about your personal relationships, your diet, your emotional well-being, and your job. The treatment may involve a host of dietary changes, stress-relieving exercises, or herbal remedies. An Ayurvedic doctor may use the tongue to diagnosis the same liver imbalance, but the approach is the same. You'll be asked about your diet, lifestyle, work habits, and so on. In other words, these practitioners do not view the body as separate from the self. And to a non-Western healer, who we are depends on our individual personalities and our societal roles; whom we marry, where we work, and how we feel about those things are just as important as our visual problems.

One of the most ancient forms of healing involves energy healing, which can involve therapeutic touch or healing touch. Technically, these techniques are considered forms of *bio-field therapy*. Several therapies help to move or stimulate the life-force energy:

- Healing touch
- *Huna*
- *Mari-el*
- *Qi gong*
- *Reiki*
- *Shen* therapy
- Therapeutic touch

An energy healer will use his or her hands to help guide your life-force energy. The hands may rest on the body or just close to the body, not actually touching it. Energy healing is used to reduce pain and inflammation, improve sleep patterns and appetite, and reduce stress. Energy healing, supported by the American Holistic Nurses Association, has been incorporated into conventional nursing techniques with good results. Typically, the healer will move loosely cupped hands in a symmetric fashion on your body, sensing cold, heat, or vibration. The healer's hands are then placed over areas where the life-force energy is imbalanced, in order to restore and regulate the energy flow.

12. Get a Massage

For many, stress relief is at their fingertips! Massage therapy—more technically referred to as soft-tissue manipulation—can be beneficial whether you're receiving the massage from your spouse or a massage therapist trained in any one of dozens of techniques from shiatsu to Swedish massage. In the East, massage was extensively written about in *The Yellow Emperor's Classic of Internal Medicine*, published in 2700 B.C. (the text that frames the entire Chinese medicine tradition). Chinese medicine recommends massage as a treatment for a variety of illnesses. It is out of shiatsu in the East and Swedish massage in the West that all the many forms of massage were developed. The following types of massage are among the most widely practiced:

- Deep-tissue massage
- Manual lymph drainage
- Neuromuscular massage
- Shiatsu
- Sports massage
- Swedish massage

Swedish massage, the method Westerners are used to experiencing, was developed in the nineteenth century by a Swedish doctor and poet, Per Henrik, who borrowed techniques from ancient Egypt, China, and Rome. Swedish-inspired massage works on physiological principles: relaxing muscles to improve blood flow throughout connective tissues, which ultimately strengthens the cardiovascular system.

Shiatsu-inspired massage focuses on balancing the life-force energy. The massage therapist in this case works to *unblock* trapped energy in various parts of your body.

While the philosophies and styles differ in each tradition, the common element is the same: to mobilize the natural healing properties of the body, which will help it maintain or restore optimal health.

No matter what kind of massage you have, the therapist uses numerous gliding and kneading techniques, along with deep circular movements and vibrations, which relax muscles, improve circulation, and increase mobility. These manipulations are known to help relieve stress and often muscle and joint pain. In general, massage can provide a variety of benefits: improved circulation, improved lymphatic system, faster recovery from musculoskeletal injuries, soothed aches and pains, reduced edema (water retention), and reduced anxiety.

In fact, a number of employers cover massage therapy on their health plans. Massage is becoming so popular that the number of licensed massage therapists enrolled in the American Massage Therapy Association has grown from 1,200 in 1983 to more than 38,000 today. To find a licensed massage therapist, see the resources listed at the back of this book.

13. Consider a Chiropractor

The word *chiropractic* comes from the Greek *chiro* and *praktikos*, which means "done by hand." This tradition was perfected in the late 1800s by Daniel David Palmer of Port Perry, Ontario. He was a self-taught healer who eventually founded a practice in Iowa. He believed that all drugs were harmful, and his theory was that disease is caused by vertebrae impinging on spinal nerves.

Chiropractors believe that the brain sends energy to every organ along the nerves that run through the spinal cord. When the vertebrae get displaced through stress, poor posture, and so on, this can block or interfere with normal nerve transmission. To cure disease in the body, the chiropractor must remove blockages through adjustments — quick thrusts, massages, and pressures along your spinal column, which move the vertebrae back to normal positions.

Sometimes adjustments involve manipulating the head and extremities (elbows, ankles, knees). This is mostly done by hand, but chiropractors may use special devices to aid them in treatment. In addition, a chiropractor will take your medical history and do a general physical exam. A chiropractor may also x-ray your spine to look for malalignments.

14. Discover Osteopathic Manipulation

Osteopathic manipulation is a hands-on healing technique utilized by an osteopathic practitioner. This involves many of the same kinds of hands-on diagnostic approaches used by a medical doctor (pressing various points to gauge whether there's pain, difficulty breathing, etc.). It also involves much more attention to your posture and gait (the way you walk), overall flexibility and mobility, and straightness of the spine. An osteopath will carefully examine your skin, too, looking for fluid retention, muscular changes, temperature variations, and tenderness. The osteopath will then use hands-on healing techniques to manipulate and stimulate muscles to improve circulation. This may be combined with standard medical treatment in certain cases, but osteopathic manipulation tends to work well to relieve the physical symptoms of stress. One of the most common forms of osteopathic manipulation is *postural drainage*, a technique for mechanically unplugging fluid blocks in the body to promote blood circulation.

15. Consider Pressure-Point Therapies

Pressure-point therapies involve using the fingertips to apply pressure to pressure points on the body. The pressure is believed to help reduce stress, pain, and other physical symptoms of stress or other ailments. Among the various kinds of pressure-point therapies, the best known are acupuncture, reflexology (see pages 32 and 33), and shiatsu.

Acupuncture

Acupuncture is an ancient Chinese healing art that aims to restore the smooth flow of life energy (qi) in your body. Acupuncturists believe that your qi can be accessed from various points on your body, such as your ear. Each point is also associated with a specific organ or part of the phyche. Depending on your physical health, an acupuncturist will use a fine needle on a very specific point to restore qi to various organs. Each of the roughly two thousand points on your body has a specific therapeutic effect when stimulated.

Acupuncture apparently stimulates the release of endorphins. This explains its effectiveness at reducing stress, anxiety, pain, and other symptoms.

Other pressure-point therapies similar to acupuncture include *jin shin jyutsu* and *jin shin do*.

Reflexology

Dr. William Fitzgerald, an American ear, nose, and throat specialist who talked about reflexology as "zone therapy," developed western reflexology. But in fact, reflexology is practiced in several cultures, including those of Egypt, India, Africa, China, and Japan. In the same way as the ears

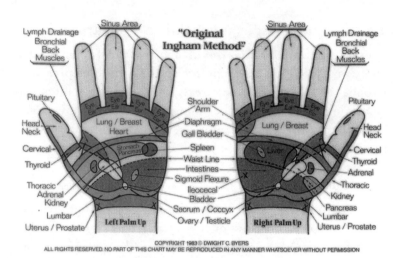

Foot and hand charts reprinted with permission from Byers, Dwight C., *Better Health with Foot Reflexology: The Original Ingham Method* (1997: Ingham Publishing, St. Petersburg). To purchase your own wallet-sized card, go to www.reflexology-usa.net.

are maps to the organs, with valuable pressure points that stimulate the life force, the feet play the same role in reflexology. A reflexologist views the foot as a microcosm of the entire body. Individual reference points or reflex areas on the foot correspond to all major organs, glands, and other parts of body. By applying pressure to certain parts of the feet, hands, and even ears, reflexologists can ease pain and tension and restore the body's life-force energy.

Like most Eastern healing arts, reflexology aims to release the flow of energy through the body along its various pathways. When this energy is trapped for some reason, illness can result. When the energy is released, the

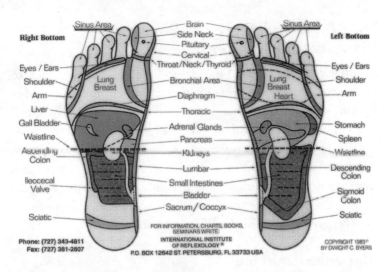

Foot and hand charts reprinted with permission from Byers, Dwight C., *Better Health with Foot Reflexology: The Original Ingham Method* (1997: Ingham Publishing, St. Petersburg). To purchase your own wallet-sized card, go to www.reflexology-usa.net.

body can begin to heal itself. Applying pressure to a specific area of the foot stimulates the movement of energy to the corresponding body part.

Shiatsu

Shiatsu massage (see Item 12) also involves using pressure points. A healer using shiatsu will travel the length of each energy pathway (also called a meridian), applying thumb pressure to successive points along the way. The aim is to stimulate acupressure points while giving you some of the healer's own life energy. In barefoot shiatsu, the healer uses the foot instead of the hand to apply pressure.

16. Stand and Deliver: Postural Reeducation Strategies

Another popular form of hands-on healing is using touch to guide your body into better posture and alignment, similar in some ways to chiropractic healing (see Item 13). Postural reeducation, as it is called, involves using touch. By learning better posture, coordination, and balance, you can relieve structural and functional stress. Three of the most common postural reeducation methods used in North America are the Alexander technique, the Feldenkrais method, and Trager psychophysical integration.

Alexander Technique

The Alexander technique involves the repositioning of the head, neck, and shoulders. Developed by Shakespearean actor Frederick Matthias Alexander (1869–1955), it involves being verbally guided into better posture and alignment through exercises that may involve lying, sitting, standing, or walking. At the same time, you'll be instructed about areas that have posture-related tension. By avoiding certain movements, you can greatly decrease back pain or back problems, improve overall health, and improve your mental health through better focus and more patience.

Feldenkrais Method

Physicist Moshe Feldenkrais believed that movement, thought, speech, and feelings are a reflection of self-image. He argued that when people become aware of their habits related to motion, they can learn to move more easily and gracefully, resulting in improved self-image and better health. The Feldenkrais method combines verbal guidance and gentle touch to make you aware of customary movement patterns and possible alternatives. More graceful and aware movements can improve stress-related symptoms and overall health.

Trager Method

Developed by Milton Trager, M.D. (1908–1997), this therapy is often called the the Trager approach, and it involves learning the joy of movement. Trager was born with a congenital spinal deformity, and through this method, he developed an athletic and graceful body. Healers use their hands to direct you through exercises involving bouncing, rocking, shaking, compression, and elongation. This approach assumes that using and moving your body—in all ways it *can* be moved—will improve mind-set, flexibility, and overall health, as well as reduce stress-related tension.

17. Try Rolfing: Structural Integration

Developed by Ida Rolf, a biophysicist, Rolfing involves realigning bad posture that has been caused by trauma or injury. A healer using the Rolfing technique will coax bones and muscles into their proper alignment by using the thumbs, fingers, and elbows to deliver a sliding pressure to the affected area. Rolfing can cause some discomfort because it involves stretching the deep tissues sufficiently to bring the head, torso, pelvis, legs, and feet into alignment. But the results can be rewarding; this technique can greatly alleviate stress.

18. Know Where to Find (and How to Use) Hands-On Healers

If you're interested in trying out one of the hands-on healing techniques, contact your family doctor or chiropractor for a referral. Naturopathic physicians also are a good source, and you can consult the resource list at the back of this book for specific organizations that can refer you to practitioners in your area. Another good way of locating these practitioners is to apply the "hairdresser rule": ask friends and family members who have had good experiences with any of these techniques.

When you find the practitioner in the discipline that interests you, tell him or her about any medical conditions you have and medications you're taking. There is evidence that some of these techniques could worsen certain medical conditions. So if you have inflamed or infected tissue, an infectious disease, a serious heart condition, or are undergoing treatment for cancer, consult your doctor before undergoing any of these therapies. For many of these healing techniques, the benefits have not been proved by standard Western studies. When researching alternative therapies, most Western researchers don't know enough about the therapies to design proper studies. And many of these ancient disciplines just don't lend themselves well to Western-style research, such as double-blind controlled studies. Besides limited proof of benefits, alternative and complementary medicine has possible risks that you should be aware of:

- Since no advisory board or set of guidelines governs non-Western practitioners, the alternative industry attracts quacks and charlatans.

- Costs for some therapies can be prohibitive.

- Academic credentials are all over the map in many of these industries. Beware humbugs.

19. Learn to Give (and Receive) a Proper Back Rub

How many times have you asked someone for a back rub, only to be completely disappointed by poor technique? Now you can hand your back rubber this page. You can also show the back rubber the right way to do it, by reciprocating the favor.

Step one: Using the heels of your hands, do a long stroke, starting from the buttocks and following the length of the spine (both sides of the spine).

Step two: At the shoulders, use your thumbs to form small deep circles, starting in the interior part of the shoulder blades, moving up the spine into the base of the head, then down to the small of the back.

Step three: At the base of the head, press your forefinger and middle finger into the furrows.

Repeat these steps until the recipient is relaxed.

20. Learn to Work Your Own Pressure Points

You can relieve stress with your own hands, too. Here are some simple pressure-point exercises you can try:

- With the thumb of one hand, slowly work your way across the palm of the other hand, from the base of the baby finger to the base of the index finger. Then rub the center of your palm with your thumb. Push on this point. This will calm your nervous system. Repeat this, using the other hand.

- To relieve a headache, grasp the flesh at the base of one thumb with the opposite index finger and thumb. Squeeze gently and massage the tissue in a circular motion. Then, pinch each fingertip. Switch to the other hand.

- For general stress relief, find sore pressure points on your feet and ankles. Gently press your thumb into them, and work each sore point. The tender areas are signs of stress in particular parts of your body. By working them, you're relieving the stress and tension in various organs, glands, and tissues. You can also apply pressure with bunched and extended fingers, the knuckles, and the heel of the hand, or with a gripping motion.

- Also use the preceding technique for self-massage on the hands, looking for tender points on the palms and wrists.

- Use the same technique to self-massage the ears. Feel for tender spots on the flesh of the ears, and work them with vigorous massage. Normally, within about four minutes, the ears will get very hot.

PART THREE

Antistress Herbs and Nutrients

21. Calm Your Nerves with Herbs

There are a variety of *nerve herbs* available over the counter at most drugstores or natural-health stores. Saying that an herb is *nervine* means that it has a positive effect on the nervous system. It could be toning, relaxing, stimulating, antidepressant, or analgesic. Many people find the following herbs and dietary supplements helpful in combating emotional symptoms (irritability, anxiety, sleeplessness, and mild to moderate depression) that stress can create.

- *Saint-John's-wort.* Also known as *Hypericum*, this has been used as a sort of *nerve tonic* in folk medicine for centuries. Studies have shown that Saint-John's-wort can successfully treat mild to moderate depression and anxiety. The American Psychiatric Association has endorsed it as a first line of treatment for depression. In Germany and other parts of Europe, Saint-John's-wort outsells Prozac prescriptions. Since it was introduced into North

America in the early 1990s, millions of North Americans have successfully used Saint-John's-wort to treat their depression. In the United States, sales of Saint-John's-wort and other botanical products reached an estimated $4.3 billion in 1998, according to *Nutrition Business Journal.* The advantages of Saint-John's-wort are that it has minimal side effects, can be mixed with alcohol, is nonaddictive, and doesn't require increases in dosage as antidepressants do. You can go on and off Saint-John's-wort as you wish, without any problem. It helps you sleep and dream, yet it has no sedative effect and, in fact, enhances your alertness.

- *Kava root.* From the black-pepper family, another popular herb is kava (*Piper methysticum*), which has been a popular herbal drink in the South Pacific for centuries. Kava, which grows on the islands of Polynesia, is known to have an antidepressant effect that calms nerves and eases stress, fatigue, and anxiety. Kava can also help alleviate migraine headaches and menstrual cramps. In placebo-controlled studies conducted by the National Institute of Mental Health, kava significantly relieved anxiety and stress, without the problem of dependency or addiction to the herb. Kava should not be combined with alcohol, because it can make the effects of alcohol more potent. Also, you should check with your doctor before you combine kava with any prescription medications.

- *SAM-e.* Pronounced "Sammy," this is another natural compound shown to help alleviate anxiety and mild depression. SAM-e stands for S-adenosylmethionine, a compound made by your body's cells. Since it was introduced in the United States in March 1999, more people have purchased SAM-e than Saint-John's-wort. SAM-e has also been shown to help relieve joint pain and to improve liver function, which makes it popular for the people suffering from arthritis as well. Studies done in Italy during the 1970s documented SAM-e's effectiveness as an antidepressant; recent U.S. studies confirm these results. Some people have reported hot, itchy ears as a side effect.

- *Gamma-aminobutyric acid (GABA).* This amino acid is supposedly an antianxiety agent. It may also help you to fall asleep if you suffer from sleeplessness.

- *Inositol.* This naturally occurring antidepressant is present in many foods, such as vegetables, whole grains, milk, and meat. It should be available over the counter.

- *Dehydroepiandrosterone (DHEA).* This hormone is produced by the adrenal glands, but production declines as we age. Studies have linked DHEA to improved moods and memory.

- *Melatonin.* Another hormone, melatonin improves sleep and helps reset the body's natural clock.

- *Phosphatidylserine (PS).* This is a phospholipid, a substance that feeds brain-cell membranes. Some studies show it has natural antidepressant qualities.

- *Tetrahydrobiopterin (BH4).* This substance activates enzymes that control serotonin, noradrenaline, and dopamine levels, which are all important for stable moods. Some studies show BH4 is an effective natural treatment for depression.

- *Phenylethylamine (PEA).* This nitrogen-containing compound occurs in small quantities in the brain. Studies show it works as a natural antidepressant.

- *Rubidium.* This element occurs naturally in our bodies and belongs to the same family as lithium, potassium, and sodium. Studies show that it can work as an antidepressant.

- *Ginkgo.* A plant used to treat a variety of ailments, ginkgo is a common herb in Chinese medicine. It can improve memory, and some studies show that it can boost the effectiveness of antidepressant medications.

- *Valerian root.* Similar to kava root in that it works as an antianxiety agent, as well as combating insomnia. A combination of valerian root with passionflower, oatstraw, or *chamomile* is very relaxing and toning, and it makes you feel restored.

- *Ginseng.* This herbal supplement helps you adapt better to stress (physical or psychological). It is also considered to boost the immune system.

- *Astragalus.* Similar to ginseng, this Chinese herb helps you adapt to stress by strengthening the immune system.

Flower Power

Flowers from the following trees can help strengthen your emotions: aspen, willow, holly, larch, mustard, pine, beech, elm, and white chestnut. They can be found at most health-food stores as supplements or in teas.

22. Consider Aromatherapy

Essential oils, derived from plants (mostly herbs and flow-ers), can do wonders to relieve stress naturally. Many essen-tial oils are known for their calming and antidepressant effects. The easiest way to use essential oils is in a warm bath—simply drop a few drops of the oil into the bath and then sit and relax in it for about ten minutes. The oils can also be inhaled (put a few drops in a bowl of hot water, lean over with a towel over your head, and breathe), diffused (using a lamp ring or a ceramic diffuser), or sprayed into the air as a mist.

The following essential oils are known to have calming, sedative, and/or antidepressant effects: ylang-ylang, neroli, jasmine, orange blossom, cedarwood, lavender (a few drops on your pillow will also help you sleep), chamomile, mar-joram, geranium, patchouli, rose, sage, clary sage, and sandalwood.

The following scents are considered stimulating and ener-gizing: lemon, grapefruit, peppermint, rosemary, and pine.

23. Take These to Heart

If stress is causing you to experience heart palpitations or you're concerned about the effects of stress on your heart, you may want to add the following nutrients to your diet. These are good for strengthening or nourishing the heart:

- *Wheat germ oil.* Take 1 or more tablespoons (15 ml) daily.

- *Vitamin E oil.* Take 1 or more tablespoons (15 ml) daily.

- *Flaxseed oil.* Flaxseed (*Linum usitatissimum*), also known as linseed, is considered the best heart oil— but only if it is absolutely fresh and taken uncooked. The recommended amount is 1 to 3 teaspoons (5 to 15 ml) of flaxseed oil first thing in the morning. You may grind the seeds and sprinkle them on cereals or salads, or soak them in water and drink.

- *Borage or black currant seed.* Other heart-protective oils can be found in the freshly pressed oils of borage seed or black currant seed.

- *Plantain, lamb's-quarter, and amaranth.* Each of these plants contains essential fatty acids.

- *Hawthorn berry tincture.* Take 25 to 40 drops of the berry tincture up to four times a day.

- *Seaweed*

- *Carotene-rich foods.* Look for bright-colored fruits and vegetables. The richer the color, the richer they are in carotene.

- *Garlic, Knoblauch.* The greatest heart benefits come from eating garlic raw, but you can also purchase deodorized caplets.

- *Lemon balm.* Steep a handful of fresh leaves in a glass of white wine for an hour or so, and drink the wine with dinner. Or make lemon balm vinegar to use on your salads.

- *Dandelion root tincture.* Use 10 to 15 drops with meals.

- *Ginseng* (Panax quinquefolius). Chew on the root, or use 5 to 40 drops of tincture.

- *Motherwort (Leonurus cardiaca).* Use a tincture of the flowering tops, 5 to 15 drops several times a day as needed.

The following herbs are good for calming the heart:

- *Rose flower essence*
- *Hawthorn (Crataegus).* Try 25 to 40 drops up to four times a day. It is slow-acting, requiring about a month of use before you see results.
- *Motherwort tincture.* Use 10 to 20 drops with meals and before bed or 25 to 50 drops for immediate relief.
- *Valerian root.* Take as a tea or tincture.
- *Gingerroot.* Take as a tea, served hot or cold.
- *Licorice root.* Chew a piece of real licorice root to slow palpitations.

24. Lower Your Risk of Heart Attack or Stroke with Herbs and Nutrients

Blood thinners, such as aspirin, can reduce the incidence of a stroke or heart attack. However, a daily spoonful of vinegar made from the leaves, buds, and/or flowers of any of the following herbs can give you the same health benefits of aspirin, while also helping calcium absorption and improving your digestion: alfalfa, birch, sweet clover, bedstraw, poplar, red clover, willow, and wintergreen.

Another blood-thinning herb is black haw (*Viburnum*). Use as a tincture. Try a 25-drop dose as needed.

Caution: Do not take blood-thinning herbs if you are bleeding heavily or require surgery.

To Lower Blood Pressure

The following supplements are believed to reduce blood pressure:

- *Hawthorn.* Use as a tincture, 10 to 20 drops three times daily.

- *Motherwort.* Use as a tincture, 10 to 20 drops three times daily.

- *Dandelion root.* As a tincture, use 10 to 15 drops with meals.

- *Potassium.* Among people who eat six portions of potassium-rich foods daily, 80 to 85 percent will reduce their need for blood-pressure-lowering medication by half or more.

- *Raw garlic.* Just ½ to 1 clove of raw garlic a day can dramatically reduce your blood pressure. Mince it raw into a variety of dishes, including eggs, rice, or potatoes.

- *Ginseng* (any amount)

- *Seaweed* (any amount)

25. Give Your Immune System a Boost

Stress lowers your resistance to disease by suppressing your immune system. The following list provides an overview of some of the best-known immune boosters, which stimulate your immune system or strengthen it to help fight diseases, including cancer:

- *Echinacea.* A flower belonging to the sunflower family, echinacea is believed to increase the number of disease-fighting cells in your immune system.

- *Essiac.* This mixture of four herbs (Indian rhubarb, sheepshead sorrel, slippery elm, and burdock root) is believed to strengthen the immune system, improve appetite, supply essential nutrients to the body, possibly relieve pain, and ultimately, prolong life.

- *Ginseng.* A root used in Chinese medicine, ginseng is believed to enhance your immune system and boost the activity of white blood cells.

- *Green tea.* This is a popular Asian tea made from a plant called *Camellia sinensis.* The active chemical in green tea, *epigallocatechin gallate* (EGCG), is believed to neutralize free radicals, which are carcinogenic. Green tea is thus considered an anticancer agent, particularly for stomach, lung, and skin cancers.

- *Iscador (mistletoe).* Iscador is made through a fermentation process, using different kinds of mistletoe, a plant known for its white berries. More popular as an antitumor treatment in Europe, iscador is believed to work by enhancing your immune system and inhibiting tumor growth.

- *Paul d'Arco (Tabeebo).* This usually comes in the form of a tea made from the inner bark of a tree called tabebuia. It's believed to act as a cleansing agent and can be used as an antimicrobial agent. This tea is also said to stop tumor growth.

- *Wheatgrass.* This grass, grown from wheatberry seeds, is rich in chlorophyll. Its juice contains over one hundred vitamins, minerals, and other nutrients and is believed to contain a number of cancer-fighting agents and immune-boosting properties.

The following herbs and spices also are said to be tumor busters: garlic, turmeric, onions, black pepper, asafetida, pippali, cumin, poppy seeds, kandathiipile, neem flowers, mananthakkali, drumstick, basil leaves, ponnakanni, and parsley.

26. Combat Digestive Disorders with Herbs and Spices

Stress can seriously interfere with digestion. The following spices can aid digestion anytime, but especially during high-stress periods:

- *Coriander* eases gases and works to tone the digestive system. Use seeds powdered or whole, or garnish food with fresh leaves (cilantro).

- *Cardamom* reduces the mucus-forming effects of dairy products. Use seeds powdered or whole.

- *Turmeric* generally improves metabolism and helps you to digest proteins. Use the root ground. (It gives dishes a yellowish color and can stain clothes and china.)

- *Black pepper* stimulates the appetite and helps you digest dairy products. Use it freshly ground.

- *Cumin* helps reduce gases and generally tones the digestive system. Use seeds whole or powdered.

- *Fennel* helps prevent gas. Chew the seeds after eating, or add them when cooking vegetables that tend to produce gas. Use the seeds whole or powdered.

- *Ginger* aids digestion and respiration. It helps to relieve gas and constipation or indigestion. Use the root fresh or dried. (**Caution:** Ginger can aggravate bleeding ulcers.)

- *Cinnamon* naturally cleanses your digestive system. Use this spice powdered or in sticks.

- *Nutmeg* helps your body absorb nutrients from food.

- *Clove* also helps your body absorb nutrients. Use whole or ground cloves.

- *Cayenne* helps to stimulate your digestive juices and is known for having a cleansing action within the large intestine. It helps to relieve that feeling of fullness after eating a heavy meal.

- *Licorice root* acts as a general digestive aid. Take 2 to 4 capsules after meals.

27. Eat Well to Reduce Stress

We now know that a variety of daily nutrients help to regulate our stress levels and our moods. For example, *tryptophan*, which is found in milk and other dairy products, helps our bodies to build neurotransmitters, such as *serotonin*.

The B vitamins are also important for mental health. Vitamin B_{12} is crucial for good general health, while other B-complex vitamins (thiamine, riboflavin, niacin, pyridoxine, pantothenic acid, and biotin) are essential for brain function, enabling you to be cognizant and alert. When you don't have enough "brain foods," you can become more prone to stress, anxiety, or depression.

The following list identifies various essential nutrients and their natural sources:

Vitamin A/beta-carotene is found in liver, fish oils, egg yolks, whole milk, and butter, beta-carotene in leafy greens and in yellow and orange vegetables and fruits. This nutrient is depleted by coffee, alcohol, cortisone, mineral oil, fluorescent lights, liver cleansing, excessive intake of iron, or a lack of protein.

Vitamin B$_6$ is found in meats, poultry, fish, nuts, liver, bananas, avocados, grapes, pears, egg yolk, whole grains, and legumes.

Vitamin B$_{12}$ is found in meats, dairy products, eggs, liver, and fish. Both B$_{12}$ and B$_6$ are depleted by coffee, alcohol, tobacco, sugar, raw oysters, and birth-control pills.

Vitamin C is found in citrus fruits, broccoli, green peppers, strawberries, cabbage, tomatoes, cantaloupe, potatoes, and leafy greens. Herbal sources are rose hips, yellow dock root, raspberry leaf, red clover, hops, nettles, pine needles, dandelion greens, alfalfa, echinacea, skullcap, parsley, cayenne, and paprika. Vitamin C is depleted by antibiotics, aspirin and other pain relievers, coffee, stress, aging, smoking, baking soda, and high fever.

Vitamin D is found in fortified milk, butter, leafy green vegetables, egg yolk, fish oils, butter, liver, skin exposure to sunlight, and shrimp. There are no herbal sources, as this vitamin is not found in plants. It is depleted by mineral oil used on the skin, frequent baths, and sunscreens with SPF 8 or higher.

Vitamin E is found in nuts, seeds, whole grains, fish-liver oils, fresh leafy greens, kale, cabbage, and asparagus. Herbal sources include alfalfa, rose hips, nettles, dang gui, watercress, dandelions, seaweeds, and wild seeds. Vitamin E is depleted by mineral oil and sulfates.

Vitamin K is found in leafy greens, corn and soybean oils, liver, cereals, dairy products, meats, fruits, egg yolk, and blackstrap molasses. Herbal sources are nettles, alfalfa, kelp, and green tea. Vitamin K is depleted by x-rays and other forms of radiation, air pollution, enemas, frozen foods, antibiotics, rancid fats, and aspirin.

Thiamine (vitamin B_1) is found in asparagus, cauliflower, cabbage, kale, spirulina, seaweeds, and citrus. Herbal sources are peppermint, burdock, sage, yellow dock, alfalfa, red clover, fenugreek, raspberry leaves, nettles, catnip, watercress, yarrow, briar rose buds, and rose hips.

Riboflavin (vitamin B_2) is found in beans, greens, onions, seaweeds, spirulina, dairy products, and mushrooms. Herbal sources are peppermint, alfalfa, parsley, echinacea, yellow dock, hops, dandelion, ginseng, dulse, kelp, and fenugreek.

Pyridoxine (vitamin B_6) is found in baked potato with skin, broccoli, prunes, bananas, dried beans and lentils, as well as in all meats, poultry, and fish.

Folic acid (B factor) is found in liver, eggs, leafy greens, yeast, legumes, whole grains, nuts, fruits (bananas, orange juice, and grapefruit juice), and vegetables (broccoli, spinach, asparagus, and brussels sprouts). Herbal sources include nettles, alfalfa, parsley, sage, catnip, peppermint, plantain, comfrey leaves, and chickweed.

Niacin (B factor) is found in a variety of grains, meats, and nuts, but especially in asparagus, spirulina, cabbage, and bee pollen. Herbal sources are hops, raspberry leaf, red clover, slippery elm, echinacea, licorice, rose hips, nettles, alfalfa, and parsley.

Bioflavonoids are found in citrus pulp and rind. Herbal sources are buckwheat greens, blue-green algae, elderberries, hawthorn fruits, rose hips, horsetail, and shepherd's purse.

Carotenes are found in carrots, cabbage, winter squash, sweet potatoes, dark leafy greens, apricots, spirulina, and seaweeds. Herbal sources include peppermint, yellow dock, uva ursi, parsley, alfalfa, raspberry leaves, nettles, dandelion greens, kelp, green onions, violet leaves, cayenne, paprika, lamb's-quarters, sage, peppermint, chickweed, horsetail, black cohosh, and rose hips.

Essential fatty acids, including *GLA*, *omega-6*, and *omega-3*, are found in safflower oil, wheat germ oil, and fatty fish. Herbal sources include all wild plants. Commercial sources are flaxseed oil, evening primrose, black currant, and borage.

Boron is found in organic fruits, vegetables, and nuts. Herbal sources are all organic weeds, including chickweed, purslane, nettles, dandelion, and yellow dock.

Calcium is found in milk and dairy products, leafy greens, broccoli, clams, oysters, almonds, walnuts, sunflower seeds, sesame seeds (including tahini), legumes, tofu, softened bones of canned fish (sardines, mackerel, and salmon), seaweed vegetables, whole grain, whey, and shellfish. Herbal sources are valerian, kelp, nettles, horsetail, peppermint, sage, uva ursi, yellow dock, chickweed, red clover, oatstraw, parsley, black currant leaf, raspberry leaf, plantain leaf and seed, borage, dandelion leaf, amaranth leaves, and lamb's-quarters. This mineral is depleted by coffee, sugar, salt, alcohol, cortisone, enemas, and too much phosphorus. Calcium and magnesium help your brain to properly transmit nerve impulses.

Chromium is found in barley grass, bee pollen, prunes, nuts, mushrooms, liver, beets, and whole wheat. Herbal sources are oatstraw, nettles, red clover, catnip, dulse, wild yam, yarrow, horsetail, black cohosh, licorice, echinacea, valerian, and sarsaparilla. Chromium is depleted by white sugar.

Copper is found in liver, shellfish, nuts, legumes, water, organically grown grains, leafy greens, seaweeds, and bittersweet chocolate. Herbal sources are skullcap, sage, horsetail, and chickweed.

Iron occurs in two forms. *Heme* iron is easily absorbed by the body; *nonheme* iron not as easily absorbed, so should be taken with Vitamin C. Heme iron is found in liver, meat, and poultry. Nonheme iron is found in dried fruit, seeds, almonds, cashews, enriched and whole grains, legumes, and green leafy vegetables. Herbal sources of iron include chickweed, kelp, burdock, catnip, horsetail, althaea root, milk thistle seed, uva ursi, dandelion leaf and root, yellow dock root, dang gui, black cohosh, echinacea, plantain leaves, sarsaparilla, nettles, peppermint, licorice, valerian, and fenugreek. Iron is depleted by coffee, black tea, enemas, alcohol, aspirin, carbonated drinks, lack of protein, and excess dairy.

Magnesium is found in leafy greens, seaweeds, nuts, whole grains, yogurt, cheese, potatoes, corn, peas, and squash. Herbal sources are oatstraw, licorice, kelp, nettle, dulse, burdock, chickweed, althaea root, horsetail, sage, raspberry leaf, red clover, valerian, yellow dock, dandelion, carrot tops, parsley, and evening primrose. Magnesium is depleted by alcohol, chemical diuretics, enemas, antibiotics, and excessive fat intake.

Manganese is found in any leaf or seed from a plant grown in healthy soil, as well as in seaweeds. Herbal sources are raspberry leaf, uva ursi, chickweed, milk thistle, yellow dock, ginseng, wild yam, hops, catnip, echinacea, horsetail, kelp, nettles, and dandelion.

Molybdenum is found in organically raised dairy products, legumes, grains, and leafy greens. Herbal sources include nettles, dandelion greens, sage, oatstraw, fenugreek, raspberry leaves, red clover, horsetail, chickweed, and seaweeds.

Nickel is found in chocolate, nuts, dried beans, and cereals. Herbal sources include alfalfa, red clover, oatstraw, and fenugreek.

Phosphorus is found in whole grains, seeds, and nuts. Herbal sources are peppermint, yellow dock, milk thistle, fennel, hops, chickweed, nettles, dandelion, parsley, dulse, and red clover. This nutrient is depleted by antacids.

Potassium is found in celery, cabbage, peas, parsley, broccoli, peppers, carrots, potato skins, eggplant, whole grains, pears, citrus fruits, and seaweeds. Herbal sources include sage, catnip, hops, dulse, peppermint, skullcap, kelp, red clover, horsetail, nettles, borage, and plantain. Potassium is depleted by coffee, sugar, salt, alcohol, enemas, vomiting, diarrhea, chemical diuretics, and dieting.

Selenium is found in dairy products, seaweeds, grains, garlic, liver, kidneys, fish, and shellfish. Herbal sources are catnip, milk thistle, valerian, dulse, black cohosh, ginseng, uva ursi, hops, echinacea, kelp, raspberry leaf, rose buds and hips, hawthorn berries, fenugreek, sarsaparilla, and yellow dock.

Silicon is found in unrefined grains, root vegetables, spinach, and leeks. Herbal sources are horsetail, dulse, echinacea, cornsilk, burdock, oatstraw, licorice, chickweed, uva ursi, and sarsaparilla.

Sulfur is found in eggs, dairy products, cabbage-family plants, onions, garlic, parsley, and watercress. Herbal sources include nettles, sage, plantain, and horsetail.

Zinc is found in oysters, other seafood, meat, liver, eggs, whole grains, wheat germ, pumpkin seeds, and spirulina.

Herbal sources include skullcap, sage, wild yam, chickweed, echinacea, nettles, dulse, milk thistle, and sarsaparilla. Zinc is depleted by alcohol and air pollution.

Carbohydrates and Stress

One of the most important factors in combating stress is
maintaining normal blood sugar levels. Many people suffer
from repeated episodes of low blood sugar, known as *hypo-
glycemia*. This is usually caused by consuming too many carbohydrates, which produce an initial rush of energy,
followed by a tremendous crash, sometimes known as *post-
prandial depression* (meaning after-meal depression). In fact,
when you're under stress or feeling depressed, it's not at all
unusual to crave simple carbohydrates, such as sugars and
sweets. The simpler the carbohydrate, the faster it breaks
down into glucose, and the faster the drop in blood sugar,
leading to a drop in mood.

If you think you suffer from low blood sugar, schedule
an appointment with a nutritionist through your primary-
care physician. Plan a diet that is based on a variety of
foods, rather than one that is mostly carbohydrates. By
increasing your intake of protein and fiber, you can help to
delay the breakdown of your food into glucose, which will
keep your blood sugar levels more stable throughout the
day.

Finally, stress can cause us to miss meals or eat on the
run, which means we're often eating high-starch foods with
very little nutrients. Instead, sit down to eat meals, and try
to rest or relax before eating. These practices can improve
digestion.

28. Avoid Overeating

On the flip side, many people overeat when under stress—
sometimes to the point of eating compulsively. The following behaviors are typical of a compulsive eater:

- Eating when not hungry
- Feeling out of control when around food—either
  trying to resist it or gorging on it
- Spending a lot of time thinking or worrying about
  food and one's weight
- Feeling desperate to try another diet that promises
  results
- Feeling self-loathing and shame
- Hating one's own body
- Being obsessed with what one can or will eat, or has
  eaten
- Eating in secret or with "eating partners"
- Appearing in public to be a professional dieter who's
  in control
- Buying cakes or pies and treating them as gifts—for
  example, having them wrapped to hide the fact that
  they're for oneself
- Feeling either out of control with food (compulsive
  eating) or imprisoned by it (dieting)
- Feeling temporary relief by not eating
- Looking forward with pleasure and anticipation to
  the time when one can eat alone
- Feeling unhappy because of one's eating behavior

Most people eat when they're hungry. But if you're a compulsive eater, hunger cues have nothing to do with when you eat. You may eat for any of the following reasons:

- To take part in a social event, including family meals or meeting friends at restaurants, where the food is the entertainment, even when you're not hungry

- To satisfy *mouth hunger*—the need to have something in your mouth, even though you're not hungry

- To prevent future hunger ("Better eat now, because later I may not get a chance")

- As a reward for enduring a bad day or bad experience, or to celebrate a good day or good experience

- Because "It's the only pleasure I can count on!"

- To quell nerves

- Because you're bored

- To reward, comfort, or protect yourself because you're "going on a diet" tomorrow (so you fear that you will be deprived later)

- Because food is your "friend"

Food addiction, like other addictions, can be treated successfully with the twelve-step program, begun in the 1930s by an alcoholic who overcame his addiction by essentially saying, "God, help me!" He found other alcoholics who were in a similar position, and through an organized, non-judgmental support system, they overcame addiction by realizing that "God" (a higher power, spirit, force, physical properties of the universe, or intelligence) *helps those who help themselves*. In other words, you have to want the help. This is the premise of Alcoholics Anonymous, the most successful recovery program for addicts.

People with other addictions have adopted the same program, using Alcoholics Anonymous and the "The 12 Steps and 12 Traditions," the founding literature for Alcoholics Anonymous. Overeaters Anonymous (OA) substitutes the phrase *compulsive overeater* for *alcoholic*, and *food* for *alcohol*. The theme of all twelve-step programs is best expressed through the Serenity Prayer, the first line being "God grant me the serenity to accept the things I cannot change, the courage to change the things I can, and the wisdom to know the difference." In other words, you can't take back the food you ate yesterday or last year, but you can stop feeling guilty and start controlling the food you eat today. Every twelve-step program also has the Twelve Traditions, which essentially are a code of conduct.

OA membership is divided into all-female and all-male groups. To join an OA program, you need only take the first step. Most people are able to do abstinence and the next two steps in a six- to twelve-month period before moving on. In an OA program, *abstinence* means three meals daily (weighed, measured, and recorded) with nothing in between except sugar-free or no-calorie beverages and sugar-free gum. The program also advises you to get your doctor's approval before starting.

Abstinence progresses one day at a time with the help of *sponsors* — recovering overeaters who have been there and who can talk you through your cravings. In addition, they will check your progress and are available to discuss your daily food intake.

29. Supplement Your Diet with Antistress Vitamins

Often when you're under stress, you're also depleted of vitamins and minerals. Most of us know the "antistress" vitamins:

- Vitamin C. The Recommended Daily Intake (RDI) is 4 to 8 g.

- The B vitamins. Of particular importance are cobalamin (vitamin B_{12}), with an RDI of 50 to 250 mcg; niacin (vitamin B_3), with an RDI of 50 to 150 mg; pyridoxine (vitamin B_6), with an RDI of 50 to 100 mg; and riboflavin (vitamin B_2), with an RDI of 50 to 100 mg. These can be found in a B-complex vitamin supplement.

You should also supplement with the following nutrients (listed alphabetically):

- Beta-carotene, 10,000 to 25,000 IU
- Bioflavonoids, 250 to 500 mg
- Biotin, 150 to 500 mcg
- Calcium, 600 to 1,000 mg
- Chromium, 200 to 400 mcg
- Copper, 2 to 3 mg
- Folic acid, 500 to 1,000 mcg
- Hydrochloric acid (with meals for chronic stress), 5 to 10 grains
- Inositol, 500 to 1,000 mg
- Iodine, 150 to 200 mcg

- Iron (especially for menstruating women), 10 to 20 mg
- L-amino acids (such as L-glutamine, L-tyrosine, L-phenylalanine, and L-tryptophan), 1,000 to 1,500 mg
- L-cysteine, 250 to 500 mg taken with vitamin C
- Magnesium, 350 to 600 mg (or in an Epsom salt bath)
- Manganese, 5 to 10 mg
- Molybdenum, 300 to 800 mg
- PABA, 50 to 100 mg
- Pancreatic enzymes, 1 to 2 tablets after meals
- Pantothenic acid (vitamin B_5), 500 to 1,000 mg
- Potassium, 300 to 500 mg
- Pyridoxal-5-phosphate, 25 to 75 mg
- Selenium, 200 to 400 mcg
- Sulfur, according to RDI from your doctor or pharmacist
- Superoxide dismutase, according to RDI for this enzyme from your doctor or pharmacist
- Thiamine (vitamin B_1), 75 to 150 mg
- Vitamin A, 7,500 to 15,000 IU
- Vitamin D, 400 IU
- Vitamin E, 400 to 1,000 IU
- Vitamin K, 200 to 400 mcg
- Water, 2 to 3 qt.
- Zinc, 30 to 60 mg

30. Avoid Stress Aggravators

If you're supplementing your diet with nutrients and trying to eat well to combat stress, try to cut down on substances that *aggravate* stress—substances that stimulate your heart and increase irritability.

Caffeine

One of the worst aggravators during stress is caffeine. It raises your blood pressure and increases the secretion of adrenaline, one of the stress hormones. The following list tells you how much caffeine some foods contain:

Coffee (5-oz. cup)

Brewed, drip method, 60 to 180 mg

Brewed, percolator, 40 to 170 mg

Instant, 30 to 120 mg

Decaffeinated, brewed, 2 to 5 mg

Decaffeinated, instant, 1 to 5 mg

Tea (5-oz. cup)

Brewed, major brands, 20 to 90 mg

Brewed, imported brands, 25 to 110 mg

Instant, 25 to 50 mg

Iced (12-oz. glass), 67 to 76 mg

Other

Caffeine-containing soft drink (6-oz. glass), 15 to
30 mg

Cocoa beverage (5-oz. cup), 2 to 20 mg

Chocolate milk (8-oz. glass), 2 to 7 mg

Milk chocolate (1-oz. serving), 1 to 15 mg

Semisweet dark chocolate (1-oz. serving), 5 to 35 mg

Baker's chocolate (1-oz. square), 26 mg

Chocolate-flavored syrup (1 serving), 4 mg

Nicotine

The nicotine left in your body after smoking also can aggravate stress. Worse, roughly half a million North Americans die of smoking-related illnesses each year. That's 20 percent of *all* deaths from *all* causes. We already know that smoking causes lung cancer. But did you know that smokers are also twice as likely to develop heart disease? A single cigarette affects your body within seconds, increasing heart rate, blood pressure, and the demand for oxygen (because of constricted blood vessels and carbon monoxide, a by-product of cigarettes). The greater the demand for oxygen, the greater the risk of heart disease.

Lesser-known long-term effects of smoking include a lowering of HDL, or good cholesterol, and damage to the lining of blood vessel walls, which paves the way for arterial plaque formation. In addition to increasing your risk for lung cancer and heart disease, smoking can lead to stroke, peripheral vascular disease, and a host of other cancers.

Just take a look at some of the things you'll gain by quitting this habit:

- Decreased risk of heart disease
- Decreased risk of cancer of the lung, esophagus, mouth, throat, pancreas, kidney, bladder, and cervix

- Lower heart rate and blood pressure
- Decreased risk of lung disease (bronchitis, emphysema)
- Relaxation of blood vessels
- Improved sense of smell and taste
- Healthier teeth
- Fewer wrinkles

How to Quit Smoking

Not everyone can quit smoking cold turkey, although it's a strategy that many have used successfully. (Some cold-turkey quitters report that keeping one package of cigarettes within reach lessens anxiety.) The symptoms of nicotine withdrawal begin within a few hours and peak at twenty-four to forty-eight hours after quitting. You may experience anxiety, irritability, hostility, restlessness, insomnia, and anger. For these reasons, many smokers turn to smoking cessation programs, which can include some of the following:

Behavioral counseling. Group or individual counseling can raise the rate of abstinence 20 to 25 percent. This approach to smoking cessation aims to change the mental processes of smoking, reinforce the benefits of nonsmoking, and teach skills to help the smoker avoid the urge to smoke.

Nicotine gum. Nicotine gum (Nicorette) is now available over the counter. It works as an aid to help you quit smoking by reducing nicotine cravings and withdrawal symptoms. Nicotine gum helps you wean yourself from nicotine by allowing you to gradually decrease the dosage until you stop using it altogether, a process that usually takes about twelve weeks. The only disadvantage of this method is that it caters to the oral and addictive aspects of smoking (rewarding the urge to smoke with a dose of nicotine).

Nicotine patch. Transdermal nicotine, known as the patch (Habitrol, Nicoderm, Nicotrol), doubles abstinence rates in former smokers. Most brands are now available over the counter. Each morning, you apply a new patch to a different area of dry, clean, hairless skin and leave it on for the day. Some patches are designed to be worn a full twenty-four hours. However, the constant supply of nicotine to the bloodstream sometimes causes vivid or disturbing dreams. You can also expect to feel a mild itching, burning, or tingling at the site of the patch when it is first applied. The nicotine patch works best when it is worn for at least seven to twelve weeks, with a gradual decrease in strength (nicotine dosage). Many smokers find it effective because it allows them to tackle the psychological addiction to smoking before they deal with physical symptoms of withdrawal.

Nicotine inhaler. The nicotine inhaler (Nicotrol inhaler) delivers nicotine orally via inhalation from a plastic tube. Its success rate is about 28 percent, similar to that of nicotine gum. It's available only by prescription in the United States and has yet to make its debut in Canada. Like nicotine gum, the inhaler mimics smoking behavior by responding to each craving or urge to smoke, a feature that has both advantages and disadvantages to the smoker who wants to get over the physical symptoms of withdrawal. The nicotine inhaler should be used for a period of twelve weeks.

Nicotine nasal spray. Like nicotine gum and the nicotine patch, the nasal spray reduces craving and withdrawal symptoms, allowing smokers to cut back gradually. One squirt delivers about one milligram of nicotine. In three clinical trials involving 730 patients, 31 to 35 percent were not smoking at six months. This compares to an average of 12 to 15 percent of smokers who were able to quit unaided. The nasal spray has a couple of advantages over the gum and the patch. First, nicotine is rapidly absorbed across the nasal membranes, providing a kick that is more like the real thing. Also, the prompt onset of action plus a flexible dosing schedule benefits heavier smokers. Because the nicotine reaches your bloodstream so quickly, nasal sprays have a greater potential for addiction than do the slower-acting gum and patch.

Alternative therapies. Hypnosis, meditation, and acupuncture have helped some smokers quit. In the case of hypnosis and meditation, sessions may be private or part of a group smoking cessation program.

Drugs That Help You Quit

The drug bupropion (Zyban) is an option for people who have been unsuccessful using nicotine replacement. The drug was originally prescribed as an antidepressant, and its use in smoking cessation was discovered by accident. Researchers knew that smokers trying to quit were often depressed, so they began experimenting with bupropion as a means to fight depression, not addiction. It reduces the withdrawal symptoms associated with smoking cessation and can be used in conjunction with nicotine replacement therapy. Researchers suspect that bupropion works directly in the brain to disrupt the addictive power of nicotine by affecting the same chemical neurotransmitters or messengers (such as dopamine) that nicotine does.

The pleasurable aspect of addictive drugs like nicotine and cocaine is triggered by the release of dopamine. Smoking floods the brain with dopamine. The *New England Journal of Medicine* published the results of a study of more than 600 smokers taking bupropion. At the end of treatment, 44 percent of those who took the highest dose of the drug (300 mg) were not smoking, compared to 19 percent of the group who took a placebo. By the end of one year, 23 percent of the 300 mg group and 12 percent of the placebo group were still smoke-free. Using Zyban with nicotine replacement therapy seems to improve the quit rate a bit further. Four-week quit rates from the study were 23 percent for placebo, 36 percent for the patch, 49 percent for Zyban, and 58 percent for the combination of Zyban and the patch.

Avoiding Environmental Tobacco Smoke

You don't have to smoke to suffer from the effects of nicotine. Environmental tobacco smoke (ETS) causes health problems in nonsmokers. You can reduce the impact of this stress on yourself and others by taking some of these actions to avoid or help ban ETS:

- Stop patronizing restaurants, bars, cafes, or similar businesses that allow smoking. Write to them to say they are losing your business for that reason. (If you really love the food, suggest smoking sections in a separately ventilated enclosure.)

- Write letters to the editor, naming names and identifying a particular smoke-filled restaurant or other business. State your reasons for not patronizing the business. Negative press works wonders!

- Make a point of congratulating restaurants, bars, cafes, or smaller businesses on creating smoke-free environments. Write letters, naming names to create positive press for their efforts.

If you live with a smoker or are smoking in your home, here are some ways to avoid ETS:

- Stop smoking inside the home. If you must smoke, go outdoors.

- Create a separate smoking room with its own ventilation system and air seals to keep the smoke out of the rest of the house.

- Install a more effective ventilation system with a supply of outside air and a special filter called a particulate filter.

PART FOUR

Inner and Outer Antistress Workouts

31. Get Moving

Reports from the United States show that one out of three American adults is overweight, a sign of growing inactivity. What's the definition of *sedentary*? Not moving! If you have a desk job or spend most of your time at a computer, in your car, or watching television, you are a sedentary person. If you do roughly 20 minutes of exercise less than once a week, you're relatively sedentary.

If you've been sedentary most of your life and would like to become more active, there's nothing wrong with starting by engaging in simple, even leisurely activities such as gardening, feeding the birds in a park, or doing a few simple stretches. Any step you make toward being more active is crucial.

Experts also recommend that you find a friend, neighbor, or relative to get physical with you. When your exercise plans include someone else, you'll be less apt to cancel those plans or make excuses for not getting out there.

Next, decide how often you're going to do this activity (twice, three, or four times a week? or once a day?). Try not to let two days pass without doing some exercise. If you're sedentary but otherwise healthy, aim for twenty to thirty minutes each time.

32. Make Stress-Fighting Endorphins

When you exercise, your body releases endorphins, feel-good chemicals your body naturally makes that counteract stress hormones. The best way to stimulate endorphins is through aerobic activity. But even less-intense leisure activities have the power to distract you from stress.

Aside from endorphins, aerobic activity also allows you to take more oxygen into your body, which is why it lowers the risks of so many diseases, including heart disease, stroke, and various cancers. Because the blood contains oxygen, the faster your blood flows, the more oxygen can flow to your organs. When more oxygen is in your body, you burn fat, your breathing improves, your blood pressure improves, and your heart works better. More oxygen makes our brains work better, so we feel better.

The phrase *aerobic activity* refers to activity that causes your heart to pump harder and faster, and causes you to breathe faster, which increases oxygen flow. Activities such as cross-country skiing, walking, hiking, and bicycling are all aerobic. However, even living more actively will help stimulate endorphins.

Exercise practitioners hate the terms *aerobic activity* and *aerobics program*, because these terms do not refer to what people do in their daily lives. Health promoters are replacing these terms with the phrase *active living*. That's what becoming unsedentary is all about. There are many ways you can adopt an active lifestyle. Here are some suggestions:

- If you drive everywhere, pick a parking space farther away from your destination so you can work some daily walking into your life.

- If you take public transit everywhere, get off one or two stops early so you can walk the rest of the way to your destination.

- Choose stairs more often, rather than riding escalators or elevators.

- Park at one side of the mall, and then walk to the other.

- After you eat dinner, take a stroll around your neighborhood.

- Volunteer to walk the dog.

- On weekends, find leisure activities that require strolling, such as going to the zoo, window-shopping, or visiting flea markets or garage sales.

33. Develop an Action Plan

By incorporating just one of the activities on the following lists once or twice a week, you can significantly lower stress. More-intense activities will create endorphins. Even the less-intense activities will help you find more leisure and enjoyment in your life, which also lowers stress.

More Intense	Less Intense
Skiing	Golf
Running	Bowling
Jogging	Badminton
Stair stepping or	Croquet
stair climbing	Sailing
Trampoline jumping	Swimming
Jumping rope	Strolling
Fitness walking	Stretching
Racewalking	
Aerobics classes	
Roller-skating	
Ice-skating	
Bicycling	
Weight-bearing	
exercises	
Tennis	
Swimming	

Variations on Jogging

Jogging doesn't have to be dull. Try adding some of these variations to your workout:

- After warming up with a fifteen-minute walk, alternate between walking quickly with maximum exertion for two minutes and slowing down for one minute.

- On the downhill portion of a walk or a hike, keep your heart rate up by adding lunges or squats.

- To improve your coordination and balance, vary the way you walk. Try lifting the knees as high as you can, as if marching. Alternate with a sideways "crab" walk. To strengthen the rarely used muscles of the ankles and feet, walk first on the outsides, then on the insides of your feet. Or practice walking backward.

- Use a curb for a step workout. Or climb stairs two at a time.

Water Workouts

You can also get an excellent workout in the water:

- Start by walking in water that's relatively shallow (waist- or chest-deep). Your breathing and heartbeat will determine how hard you are working. Since you'll be moving fairly slowly, pay attention to your body.

- For all-over leg toning, take fifty steps forward, fifty steps sideways in crab-like fashion, fifty steps backward, and then fifty steps to the other side.

- To tone your arms, submerge yourself to the neck, bringing the arms in and out as if clapping. The water will provide natural resistance.

- Deep-water workouts are the most difficult, because every move meets with resistance. For optimum exertion and little or no impact, wear a flotation vest and run without touching the bottom. You may also want to try buoyant ankle cuffs and Styrofoam dumbbells or kickboards for full-body conditioning in the water.

Other Activities

Above all, choose activities you enjoy. Here are more ideas to consider:

- Dancing to a rhythmic beat is a great stress-reliever as well as an excellent form of exercise. Known as *rhythmic medicine*, this kind of dancing can help people with migraine headaches, cancer, depression, high blood pressure, and other ailments.
- Hiking is another popular activity. It has the added benefit of letting you surround yourself with nature.

34. Know When to Consult a Fitness Practitioner/Trainer

Many people find it difficult to dive into a brand-new fitness routine, particularly if they have certain chronic health problems, such as diabetes, or they are taking medications that can affect their heart. In these cases, intense exercise can be dangerous. If you're just beginning to incorporate exercise into your lifestyle after many years of being sedentary, a good route is to consult with a fitness practitioner (or trainer) in the same way you might consult a nutritionist.

You can find fitness practitioners through your family doctor or through reputable fitness institutions. A fitness practitioner will plan an exercise regimen that is suited to your current physique and will slowly increase your regimen over time, as you build more stamina. Working with a fitness practitioner will also allow you to discuss your health conditions and any medications you're taking, so your activities can complement, rather than aggravate, your health conditions.

35. Practice Yoga

For many, yoga is not just about various stretches or postures—it is actually a way of life. It is part of a whole science of living known as the Ayurveda. The Ayurveda is an ancient (roughly 3,000 years old) Indian approach to health and wellness. Essentially, it divides the universe into three basic constitutions or energies known as *doshas*. The three doshas are based on wind (*vata*), fire (*pitta*), and earth (*kapha*). These doshas also govern our bodies, personalities, and activities. When your doshas are balanced, all functions well, but when they are not balanced, a state of disease (disease, as in *not at ease*) can set in. Finding the balance involves changing your diet to suit your predominant dosha. Foods are classified as kapha, vata or pitta, and we eat more or less of whatever we need for balance.

Practicing yoga is a preventive health science that involves certain physical postures, exercises, and meditation. Essentially, yoga is the exercise component of the Ayurveda. It involves relaxing meditation, breathing, and physical postures designed to tone and soothe your mental state and physical state. Most people benefit from introductory yoga classes or videos.

36. Try Deep-Breathing Exercises to Relieve Stress

Deep breathing helps to relieve a range of stress-related symptoms such as anxiety, panic attacks, and irritability. In fact, sighing and yawning are signs that that you're not getting enough oxygen in your body; the sigh or yawn is your body's way of righting the situation.

The following deep-breathing techniques are modeled after yogic breathing exercises and can calm the nervous system, relax the small arteries, and permanently lower blood pressure:

- *Abdominal breathing.* Lie down on a mat or on your bed. Take slow, deep, rhythmic breaths through your nose. When your abdominal cavity is expanded, it means your lungs have filled completely, which is important. Then, slowly exhale completely, watching your abdomen collapse again. Repeat six to ten times. Practice this morning and night.

- *Extended abdominal breathing.* This is a variation on abdominal breathing. When your abdomen expands with air, try three more short inhalations. It's akin to adding those last drops of gas to your tank when your tank is full. Then, when you exhale in one long breath, don't inhale yet. Take three more short exhales.

- *Abdominal lift.* Stand with feet at about shoulder width, bend the knees slightly, bend forward, exhale completely, and brace your hands above the knees. Then lift the abdomen upward while holding your exhalation. Your abdomen should look concave. Stand erect again, and inhale just before you feel the urge to gasp. Greer Childers, in her video *Body Flex*, demonstrates this technique very well.

- *Rapid abdominal breathing.* This is abdominal breathing done fast so it feels as though your inhalations and exhalations are forceful and powerful. Try this for twenty-five to one hundred repetitions. Each breath should last only a second or so, compared to the ten to twenty seconds involved in regular deep abdominal breathing.

- *Alternate-nostril breathing.* Hold one nostril closed, inhaling and exhaling deeply. Then alternate nostrils. This is often done prior to meditation, and it is thought to balance the left and right sides of the brain.

37. Meditate for Stress Relief

Meditation simply requires you to *stop thinking* (about your life, problems, etc.) and just *be.* To do this, people usually find a relaxing spot or sit quietly and breathe deeply for a few minutes. Going for a nature walk, playing golf, listening to music, reading inspiring poetry or prose, gardening, listening to silence, and listening only to the sounds of your own breathing are all forms of meditation. These are just a few activities that can be meditative:

- Walking or hiking
- Swimming
- Running or jogging
- Gardening
- Golf
- Music appreciation (listening, dancing, etc.)
- Reading for pleasure
- Walking your dog
- Practicing breathing exercises (see Item 36)
- Practicing stretching exercises (see Item 39)
- Practicing yoga or qi gong (see Items 35 and 38)

38. Try Qi Gong Exercises

Every morning, all over China, people of all ages gather at parks to do their daily qi gong exercises. Pronounced "chee gong," these are exercises that help get your life-force energy flowing and unblocked. (See Item 11 for more about the life-force energy.) The word *qi* means vitality, energy, and life force; the word *gong* means practice, cultivate, refine. Qi gong is similar to tai chi, except it allows for greater flexibility in routine.

Qi gong is modeled after movements in wildlife (such as birds or animals), as well as trees and other things in nature. The exercises have a continuous flow, rather than the stillness of a posture seen in yoga. Using the hands in various positions to gather in the qi, move the qi, or release the qi is one of the most important aspects of qi gong movements.

One of the first groups of qi gong exercises you might learn is the seasons—fall, winter, spring, summer, and late summer. (There are five seasons here.) These exercises look like a dance with precise, slow movements.

The Chinese believe that practicing qi gong balances the body and improves physical and mental well-being. These exercises push the life-force energy into the various meridian pathways that correspond to organs. It is the same map used in pressure-point healing (see Item 15). Qi gong improves oxygen flow and enhances the lymphatic system.

The best way to learn qi gong is through a qualified instructor. You can generally find qi gong classes through the alternative healing community. Check health food stores and other centers that offer classes such as yoga or tai chi. Qi gong is difficult to learn from a book or video. An instructor is best.

39. Stretch to Relieve Stress

Stretching improves muscle blood flow, oxygen flow, and digestion. The natural desire to stretch exists for those reasons.

The following stretches will help relieve stress and improve tranquility:

- While sitting or standing, raise your arms above your head. Keep the shoulders relaxed, and breathe deeply for five seconds. Release, and repeat five times.

- Gently raise your shoulders in an exaggerated shrug. Breathe deeply and hold for ten seconds. Relax, and repeat three times.

- Sit cross-legged on the floor, with spine straight and neck aligned. Focus on your breath, letting it gently fill the diaphragm and the back of the rib cage. On the inhalation, say, "so"; on the exhalation, say, "hum." Voicing the breath in this manner will keep you focused and relaxed. Continue with "so-hum" until you feel at ease. (This is the lotus position.)

- Kneel on your heels. Bring your forehead to the floor in front of you. Breathe into the back of the rib cage, feeling the stretch in your spine. Hold as long as it's comfortable.

- Stand tall, and find a point across the room at which to focus your gaze. Place the heel of one foot on the opposite inner thigh. Float your arms upward until your palms are touching. Breathe deeply, and hold for five seconds. Release, and repeat on the other side.

- Lie on your back with palms facing upward, feet turned gently outward. Focus on the movement of breath throughout your body.

- Lie on your belly, with arms at your sides. Bend your legs at the knees, and bring your heels in toward your buttocks. Reach back and take hold of the right, then the left ankle. If you're having a hard time maintaining this position, flex your feet. Inhale, raising the upper body as far off the floor as possible. Lift your head, completing the arch. Your knees should remain as close together as possible (tying them together might help). Breathe deeply, and hold for ten to fifteen seconds.

40. Try Antistress Postures to Improve Digestion

Since stress can badly aggravate digestion, the following antistress postures may help:

- *Locust.* Lie on your belly with your arms folded beneath you, palms pressed in to your body. Extend both legs until they lift up and off the floor. Keep the toes pointed. Release.

- *Cobra (upward-facing dog).* Lie on your belly with your palms down and adjacent to your shoulders. Slowly raise your upper body, lifting all but the lower abdomen toward the ceiling. Breathe deeply. Release.

- *Fish.* Lie on your back. Place your hands under your sitting bones, palms pressed in to the floor, feet flexed. Gently roll one, then the other shoulder

inward, shortening the distance between your
shoulder blades (your chest will naturally arch
upward). Breathe, lengthening your abdominals and
rib cage. Release.

- *Squat.* Stand with your feet parallel to your hips.
  Slowly squat, making sure your weight is forward.
  You may need to practice a few times before you can
  do this comfortably. (Squatting this way twice a day
  is recommended as an aid for constipation.)

- *Knee to chest—one leg.* Lie on your back on the floor.
  Bend one knee, and bring it in to the chest. Hug the
  leg, and slowly bring it toward your abdomen. Hold
  for a count of ten. Relax, and repeat with the other
  leg.

- *Knee to chest—both legs.* This is the same as the one-leg
  version, only you bring both legs to the chest and
  hug them with both arms, bringing them gently
  toward your abdomen. Hold them there for a count
  of ten. Then relax and repeat.

PART FIVE

Self-Care

41. Get More Sleep

Sleep deprivation is chronic in our culture. In the United States, a National Sleep Foundation survey revealed that two out of three people get less than the recommended eight hours of sleep per night; of that group, one out of three gets less than six hours of sleep. Sleep deprivation is one of the chief aggravators of stress. Lack of sleep increases levels of *cortisol*, a stress hormone. Sleep deprivation affects the immune system (depleting certain cells needed to destroy viruses and cancerous cells), promotes the growth of fat instead of muscle, and may speed up the aging process.

Cortisol is released by the adrenal gland in response to stress. It essentially is an *alertness* hormone that makes you take action. This is what causes you to be alert in important meetings, helping you close the sale or deal. The hormone will subside as the stressful event passes. Normally, cortisol declines before sleep as a way of preparing the body for the resting state. Conversely, cortisol increases in the morning to make you more alert.

A common reason people cut down on sleep is to make time for a workout before the day begins. It's not unusual for many to rise at 5:00 A.M. in order to get exercise. This, according to sleep experts, only compromises health and increases stress. The damage from sleep deprivation may cancel out the benefits of the exercises discussed in the previous section (Items 31 to 40).

Sleep involves two phases: rapid eye movement (REM) and non–rapid eye movement. REM sleep, researchers believe, is when we dream, an important component of mental health. Non-REM sleep is our deepest sleep. During this phase, the body resets various hormones and replenishes energy stores.

Roughly 50 percent of people diagnosed with depression get too much REM sleep and not enough deep sleep, the replenishing sleep. According to a study done at the University of Westminster in London, stress levels are actually lower in people who wake up later than 7:21 A.M.

One way to find more sleep is to schedule nap times. Napping after work for a couple of hours (or during the day if you work from home) can dramatically improve sleep deprivation. Avoiding alcohol and caffeine before bedtime also can help. In addition, the calming herbs discussed in Items 21 to 30 may aid sleep.

42. Get Creative

Creativity can dramatically lower stress levels, too. Creative activities include art in all its forms: words, fine arts, visual arts, healing arts, performing arts, hobbies, or sports. Writing — particularly in the form of journaling or writing

poetry or letters — is a stress buster. A recent study published in the *Journal of the American Medical Association*
reported that people suffering from chronic ailments such
as asthma or arthritis felt better when they wrote about
their ailments.

A few years ago, Oprah Winfrey used her influence to
get her viewers to begin daily journaling or diary writing.
Oprah advocated journaling because of the empowerment
it can give to those of us who are otherwise without voice
or expression. Using her own creativity to enable others,
she has resold the idea of journaling in an age where few
people take the time to sit down and be still with their
thoughts. Oprah has taken journaling one step further by
encouraging people to begin *gratitude journaling*, a process of
thinking about what, in our lives, we are thankful for, then
writing down those thoughts. This influence of Oprah, who
is a firm believer in literacy, may also give courage and the
joy of self-expression to many who once might have been
afraid to write because of low education levels. For people
who do not feel they are creative or artistic, journaling is an
opportunity to express feelings and passions.

Another successful woman, Martha Stewart, offers "creative rescue" to millions through her *lifestyle arts*. She is
essentially the mountain that comes to Mohammed. Martha
offers some good ideas for beautifying our days and rou-
tines. And when she packages her ideas as *Martha Stewart
Living*, the words invite us to come back to life and feel the
little things (which she'll tell you is good), even if it's just to
wake up and smell fresh coffee or to taste homemade sor-
bet. She offers thousands of creative tips through her program, magazine, and website.

43. Try Feng Shui

Feng shui (pronounced "fung shway") is the ancient practice of creating energy and harmony through your environmental surroundings (landscaping, interior design, architecture). These efforts can also help reduce your stress. Feng shui is said to reduce blood pressure and adrenaline levels.

People tend to think of feng shui as something that can bring wealth (as in money corners) or romance (as in hanging certain items over the bed), but this is in fact not what authentic feng shui consultants look for. Harmony has many elements. Where you live, how you live, and a host of other geographic surroundings can all affect how to arrange your environment. Feng shui consultants will assess the following elements:

- *Home entrance.* How is it lit? What do you see — flowers, chimes, or a stack of old newspapers?
- *Grounds.* What kinds or colors of flowers are around your home? Are there rocks or sculpture around the grounds of your home?
- *Specific areas inside your home.* Consultants will look at rooms and living spaces such as your work space or home office, kitchen, bedroom, bathroom, and so on. Placement of mirrors, pictures, plants, lamps, candles, rugs, furniture, bed, and even aquariums are all significant. For example, round mirrors or octagonal mirrors are powerful.

In general, feng shui tries to optimize the grounds surrounding your space through curvilinear and rectangular visual contours or edges that incorporate wildlife, landscaping or vegetation, or aquatic habitat. It also minimizes anything that interferes with harmony, such as signage and power lines. Inside the home, live plants, colors, lighting, and the positioning of furniture to maximize views of natural scenery are important.

44. Avoid Loneliness

Loneliness is stressful; solitude is not. Loneliness comes from a lack of truly intimate relationships with friends or family members. (In this case, intimacy refers to sharing deep feelings, fears, and so on.) This is how we unburden ourselves and relieve stress. Feeling as though you belong somewhere or feeling part of a community also can alleviate loneliness.

Here are steps you can take to create more supportive relationships in your life:

- Find some sort of social group to belong to by looking into gourmet cooking clubs, art classes, and so on. Find an activity that you're really drawn to, and chances are, you'll meet like-minded souls with whom you can form quality friendships.

- Have a couple of nice dinner parties each year. It's a way to create more intimate friendships with people who may be only acquaintances or casual friends.

- Get involved in your community. Whether it's a "not in my backyard" lobby or a community street sale, get out and meet your neighbors. Responding to community-based programs, ranging from crafts groups to yoga, is the way to find support. In fact, community outreach workers use the arts, crafts, fitness, computer classes, and so on as tools to attract people within the community who could benefit from support. What often takes place in community-based programs is a great deal of talking and sharing before, during, or after the activity. These are places where you make friends, find someone you can talk to, and most importantly, find that you're not alone.

- Volunteer. Volunteering for causes dear to your heart is a great way to meet people and feel needed. Meals on Wheels, elder-care facilities, street youth programs, and so forth all attract wonderful souls with whom you may find friendship and comfort.

- Get a dog. Dogs need to be walked, which means you'll meet other people walking their dogs. And dog owners tend to gravitate toward other dog owners. It's a great jumping-off point for meeting people. Aside from that, many studies point to the health effects of pet ownership, including lowered blood pressure and lowered incidence of heart disease. (Positive health effects can be seen with any pet.)

45. Consider Counseling

When you feel overwhelmed by stress, one of the best things you can do is to talk to a professional. Simply finding someone objective to talk to can make an enormous difference.

Types of Counselors

Most people looking for stress counseling do well with counselors or social workers, but all of the following professionals can help you manage your stress:

A *psychologist* or *psychological associate* is someone licensed to practice therapy with either a master's degree or doctoral degree. Clinical psychologists have a master of science (M.S.) or master of arts (M.A.) degree and usually work in a hospital or clinic setting but often can be found in private practice. Clinical psychologists can also hold a Ph.D. (doctor of philosophy) in psychology, an Ed.D. (doctor of education), or a Psy.D. (doctor of psychology).

A professional *social worker* has a degree in social work and meets state legal requirements. The professional degree may be a B.S.W. (bachelor of social work) and/or an M.S.W. (master of social work). Many social workers earned an M.S.W. after they completed a bachelor's degree in another discipline, and some social workers have earned a Ph.D. as well.

The designation CSW stands for Certified Social Worker, a legal title granted by the state. A designation of ACSW stands for Academy of Certified Social Workers. This is a nongovernmental credential of the National Association of Social Workers (NASW). In most states, to earn the CSW, a social worker must pass an exam following graduation from a master's-level program. The ACSW requires two years of supervised experience following graduation from such a program.

To work as a *psychiatric nurse*, a nurse in most states must be a registered nurse (R.N.) with a bachelor of science in nursing (B.S.). Most psychiatric nurses also have a master's degree in nursing. The master's degree could be either an M.A. (master of arts) or an M.S. (master of science). Psychiatric nurses receive most of their training in a psychiatric setting and may be trained to do psychotherapy.

A *counselor* has usually completed certification courses in counseling and obtained a license to practice psychotherapy. The license does not require a university degree, but many counselors have a master's degree in a related field, such as social work.

A *professional counselor* has earned a minimum of a master's degree and possesses professional knowledge and demonstrable skills in the application of mental health, psychological, and human development principles in order to facilitate human development and adjustment throughout the life span. As of January 1999, the District of Columbia and forty-four states have enacted some type of counselor credentialing law to regulate the use of titles related to the counseling profession. The designation CPC stands for Certified Professional Counselor and refers to the title granted by the state legislative process. LPC stands for Licensed Professional Counselor, the most frequently granted state statutory counselor credential. No matter what letters you see, however, it's always a good idea to ask your counselor what training he or she has had in the field of mental health.

In contrast to someone with the broader title of counselor, a *marriage and family counselor* has completed rigorous training through certification courses in family therapy and relationship dynamics, and has obtained a license to practice psychotherapy. A marriage and family counselor should have the designation MFT or AAFMT. MFTs have graduate training (a master's or doctoral degree) in marriage and family therapy and at least two years of clinical experience. Forty-one states currently license, certify, or regulate MFTs.

Styles of Therapy

A range of therapy techniques are used in stress counseling. Here are some of the most common:

Cognitive-behavioral therapy is oriented toward upbeat thinking and correcting what is referred to as *disordered thinking*. Instead of dwelling on negative thoughts, this form of therapy is based on the premise that how you think can affect how you feel. For example, if a friend cancels a lunch date with you or somebody doesn't return your phone call or E-mail, you may take it personally and assume that the person dislikes you. That thought leads you to feel bad about yourself, reinforcing feelings of low self-esteem or even self-loathing. A cognitive-behavioral therapist will ask you to consider other reasons for the cancellation or unreturned call. Perhaps the person was overwhelmed by problems that have absolutely nothing to do with you. Perhaps a last-minute deadline came up. In other words, not everything you perceive to be negative is really negative, and not everything you take personally is personal.

Ultimately, the premise of cognitive-behavioral therapy is this: If you think negative thoughts about yourself and believe you're a failure or that your life is doomed, you are more apt to be sad. On the other hand, if you think positive thoughts and believe in yourself, you are more apt to be happy. Essentially, what's past is past, and you can decide *today* to be a more positive person, which in turn can attract more positive experiences into your life. Although this approach might sound easy and a quick fix, changing your perspective on life can be powerful. However, in the midst of a depression, this may have limited success.

Interpersonal therapy is a very specific approach to therapy, based on the idea that malfunctioning relationships contribute to the emotional symptoms of stress. You and your therapist will explore current relationships and recent events that may have affected those relationships, such as loss, conflict, or change. You may also explore the roles various people are playing in your life, your expectations of those people, and their expectations of you. Your therapist works in a supporting role to help you develop better strategies to cope or negotiate with key people in your life, which in turn can help to resolve conflicts. Much of this has to do with setting reasonable expectations for relationships and looking at how you might have misinterpreted the actions of others.

Psychodynamic therapy deals with the ghosts of relationships and events from your past, the dynamics of your upbringing, and present events and relationships. Here, you will examine your thoughts, emotions, and behavior over a lifetime. Moreover, you will discuss patterns of behavior and aspects of your personality as possible sources of both internal and external conflict. Couples or groups are often involved in psychodynamic therapy. The adage "the past is history, the future a mystery, and the present a gift" works well in this context.

Evaluating a Therapist

Whatever style of therapy you choose, there are some hallmarks of good therapists. Look for a therapist who displays the following kinds of behavior:

- *Showing genuine concern.* Your therapist should demonstrate a basic concern for your welfare, the ability to empathize, and the ability to communicate that empathy.

- *Accepting your criticism.* If you get angry or critical, your therapist shouldn't take it personally and should be able to accept solid criticism in good measure. You need to feel assured that you can get angry or critical in a session without feeling your therapist will hold it against you or retaliate somehow. (However, a therapist should feel free to interpret your anger, if your criticism is not valid.)

- *Giving you reliable service and undivided attention.* Your therapist should not be frequently canceling sessions, changing sessions, taking phone calls during sessions, or using your time to discuss fees, payments, and so on. Nor should your therapist cut you off in the middle of an epiphany because "time's up." (Epiphanies, one presumes, don't happen every day; they should be respected.) That said, you shouldn't take advantage of your therapist and manipulate him or her for more time. Obviously, if a therapist cannot give you an extra minute now and then, there's a problem. But some clients overstep the boundary and continuously go over their time, which interferes with someone else's time. That's not fair, either.

- *Refraining from discussing his or her own problems.* Your therapist isn't your hairdresser. It's not tit for tat. You shouldn't be expected to listen to your therapist's personal problems during your therapy session.

- *Practicing within a code of ethics.* Your therapist should keep your sessions confidential and should not tape-record, videotape, or stage your session in front of a one-way mirror for colleagues to watch without your knowledge. Any time your session is being recorded or observed by others (which may be the case if the therapist is in training, is training someone else, or would like to consult with someone else about your case), you must have given your full consent. Otherwise, this is an indication that you cannot trust your therapist and should find help elsewhere.

46. Rule Out Biological Causes for "Burnout"

If you're suffering from fatigue and general malaise, before you attribute it to "just stress," see your doctor and be sure to rule out these biological causes:

- Chronic fatigue syndrome
- Thyroid disease
- Sleep disorders (such as sleep apnea or narcolepsy)
- Side effects from any medications you're taking
- Hepatitis
- Seasonal depression
- Digestive disorders
- Obesity-related fatigue
- Lyme disease

- Sexually transmitted diseases, including HIV or syphilis

- Anemia (in women, often due to heavy menstrual flow)

- Allergies (Delayed symptoms of an allergic reaction can be joint aches, pains, eczema, and fatigue. Foods and environmental toxins can be classic triggers.)

The most common conditions that mimic stress-related symptoms are discussed in the following paragraphs.

Chronic Fatigue Syndrome

The term *chronic fatigue syndrome* refers to a collection of ill-health symptoms (not just one or two), the most identifiable of which are fatigue and flu-like aches and pains. An official definition of chronic fatigue syndrome (CFS) was first published in the *Annals of Internal Medicine* in 1994. The Centers for Disease Control and Prevention (CDC) have since published official symptoms of CFS, too. Although many physicians feel the following list of symptoms is limiting and requires some expansion for accuracy, as of this writing, the official defining symptoms of CFS have two parts:

First, there is an unexplained fatigue that is "new." In other words, you've previously felt fine and have only noticed in the last six months or so that you're always fatigued, no matter how much rest you get. The fatigue is also debilitating for you; you're not as productive at work, and it interferes with normal activities that may be social, personal, or academic. You've also noticed poor memory or concentration, which affects your activities and performance, too.

In addition to this fatigue, a person with CFS has had four or more of the following conditions for a period of at least six months:

- Sore throat
- Mild or low-grade fever
- Tenderness in the neck and underarm area (where you have lymph nodes, which may be swollen, causing tenderness)
- Muscle pain (called *myalgia*)
- Pain along the nerve of a joint, without redness or swelling
- A new kind of headache, one you've never suffered from before
- Sleep that leaves you unrefreshed (a sign of insufficient amounts of non-REM sleep, as discussed in Item 41)
- Fatigue, weakness, and general unwellness for a good twenty-four hours after you've had even moderate exercise

If none of the above symptoms is responsible for your condition, you may be suffering from CFS. You also could be diagnosed with a frustrating label: *idiopathic fatigue*, which means that your fatigue is of unknown origin. This is not very helpful, and if your symptoms persist, you should find out why you don't meet CFS criteria.

Fibromyalgia

Fibromyalgia is a soft-tissue disorder that causes you to hurt all over, all the time. The condition appears to be triggered and/or aggravated by stress. If you notice fatigue and more general aches and pains, this suggests CFS. If you notice primarily joint and muscle pains, accompanied by fatigue, this suggests fibromyalgia.

Fibromyalgia is sometimes considered an offshoot of arthritis, and it's not unusual to be misdiagnosed as rheumatoid arthritis. Headaches, morning stiffness, and intolerance to cold, damp weather are common complaints with fibromyalgia. It's also common to suffer from irritable bowel syndrome or bladder problems with this disorder.

Thyroid Disease

The thyroid gland is responsible for making thyroid hormone, which drives the function of every cell in your body. If your gland is either overproducing or underproducing thyroid hormone, your energy levels and emotional responses will be greatly affected. When your thyroid gland is not making enough thyroid hormone, you suffer from *hypothyroidism*; when your thyroid gland is making too much thyroid hormone, you suffer from *hyperthyroidism*. In most cases, autoimmune diseases cause the thyroid gland to malfunction, which means that your body produces antibodies that attack the thyroid gland.

The most common autoimmune thyroid diseases are Graves' disease and Hashimoto's thyroiditis. Graves' disease causes your thyroid gland to be overactive, while Hashimoto's thyroiditis causes your thyroid gland to be underactive. Women suffer from thyroid disorders about ten times as frequently as do men, so women especially suffer from continuous and classic thyroid misdiagnosis.

Symptoms of thyroid disease come in two groups; the group of symptoms *you* suffer depends on whether you have hyperthyroidism or hypothyroidism. With hyperthyroidism, your body speeds up and becomes overworked. Your heart rate increases, you may lose weight but eat more, and you may notice excessive perspiration, an intolerance to heat, irregular menstrual periods, and diarrhea. You will also notice many of the symptoms seen in depression, such as exhaustion (from an overworked physique), insomnia, irritability, restlessness, nervousness, anxiety, and general fatigue (caused by the insomnia).

With hypothyroidism, your body slows down, creating some classic physical symptoms that include constipation, bloating and fluid retention, a decreased appetite, lack of sex drive, dry hair, dry skin, intolerance to cold temperatures, and irregular periods. The emotional symptoms of hypothyroidism are different: extreme fatigue and lethargy regardless of how much sleep you get, as well as symptoms of depression.

A simple blood test will confirm whether you are hyper- or hypothyroid. Treatment for hyperthyroidism depends on what's causing the gland to become overactive, but ultimately, your thyroid gland will probably be chemically "deadened," and you'll simply go on synthetic thyroid hormone (*levothyroxine sodium*), which replaces the natural hormone your thyroid makes. In the second scenario, synthetic thyroid hormone replenishes your diminished supply.

Seasonal Affective Disorder (SAD)

Many of the emotional symptoms of stress can be triggered by changes in seasons. A person with seasonal affective disorder (SAD) sleeps too much and eats too much (thereby gaining weight) during the winter. Then the person begins to "wake up" in the spring and can even be slightly euphoric. In short, SAD has many of the features of *hibernation*—oversleeping and storing up high fat or carbohydrates for the cold winter. It's "bear and squirrel" behavior in humans, which can be debilitating. Sometimes stress can mask SAD, or vice versa. SAD is a fairly recent diagnosis, first used in 1987.

SAD strikes people in their twenties and thirties, and is seen more in regions at higher latitudes. Living or working in areas that are light-deprived also can lead to SAD. For example, people who spend weeks or months at a time on submarines exhibit symptoms of SAD.

Light at the end of the tunnel is in sight for people with SAD—literally. If you've been diagnosed with SAD, you may be prescribed light. Often, the cure for SAD is to re-create the kind of light you'd naturally be exposed to on a nice summer's day. Sitting under your chandelier won't do. For this therapy to work, you need to sit in front of bright, full-spectrum fluorescent or incandescent lights for about 30 to 120 minutes. It's not necessary to have sunlight or sun-like light. To protect your eyes, the lights are covered with a sheer material. You can get the light you need with a *light box*. Just do whatever you like in front of these lights. You'll need to sit close—only about a foot and a half away. You need to keep your eyes open, so napping isn't a good activity. If you prefer to sleep, there is an experimental device known as a dawn simulator, which can work while you sleep. Most people start to feel better in a few days of light treatments of just 30 minutes per day.

Even this treatment has some side effects. Mild headaches or eyestrain are not unusual, and sometimes mild mania (from the production of serotonin) may occur. If you're taking a drug that makes you sensitive to bright light, you are not a good candidate for this therapy. See your doctor for information on purchasing a light box.

Bright-light therapy has also been shown to help depression that isn't necessarily SAD but is related to sleep disorders involving *circadian rhythm* (the body's natural sleep-wake cycle). In this case, light therapy during the day has been shown to help with sleep problems.

Digestive Disorders

If you suffer from digestive problems that seem related to stress, ask your doctor to rule out the following causes:

- Dietary culprits, such as food allergies, lactose intolerance, or just plain poor diet—high intake of fats and starch, and a low intake of fiber

- Intestinal bacterial, viral, or parasitic infections (possibly introduced while traveling or through sexual contact)

- Overgrowth of *C. difficile*, a common cause of infectious diarrhea

- Yeast in the gastrointestinal tract (called *candidiasis*), which is notorious for causing symptoms of irritable bowel syndrome (IBS) and can be cleared up simply by eating yogurt every day

- Side effects of medications

- Gastrointestinal disorders, such as *dysmotility*, in which the stomach muscles are not moving properly, causing bloating, nausea, and other problems

- Enzyme deficiencies (for example, the pancreas not secreting enough enzymes to break down your food)

- Serious disease such as inflammatory bowel disease or cancer

47. Pamper Yourself

Taking care of yourself means being good to yourself. Give yourself some self-TLC. You'll find this goes a long way to battle daily stresses. Here are some suggestions:

- Set aside comfort time for yourself at least once a week. Make it a ritual. It can be as simple as having coffee with your morning paper. Some other feel-good activities are going for a scenic stroll, window-shopping in a favorite neighborhood, taking a long bath, going to an open or farmers' market, or having breakfast in bed once a week. Choose any of these that will make you feel energized and loved.

- Have a very long shower each morning. Treat yourself to a shower massage, and take time each morning to massage every part of your body. Buy energizing shower gels or shower toys to use each day.

- Take a steam bath. Run the shower, and sit in your bathroom on a mat and just enjoy the steam.

- Relax in a luxurious bubble bath. Using aromatherapy to augment your bath can work wonders for relieving stress. For a spa-style bath, use mud products, dried milk powder for a milk bath, or mineral salts for aching muscles. You can enhance the bath ritual with candlelight. Use massaging oils or lotions to moisturize after the bath.

- Take a bed-rest day. Change the linens, fluff up your pillows, and prepare good reading material and a tray of favorite snacks, wine, coffee, tea, etc. Then go to bed. Spend the day as a sick day and rejuvenate.

- Plan a spa day. (Take this as a sick day if you like.) Start your day in the bath, as described earlier. Then go outside for a nice long walk. Come back inside and take an invigorating shower, scrubbing your body with a loofah scrubber or rough washcloth. Then wash your hair and put in a deep conditioning treatment. Or smooth the calluses on your feet. Start another bath with essential oils (see Item 22). Cleanse your face well, and apply your favorite facial mask. Light candles and soak, while putting a cool washcloth over your eyes. Then get back in the shower, rinse off the mask, and remoisturize your body. Wrap yourself in a towel and take a nap. (You may want to arrange in advance for a massage therapist to visit you at this point!) After your nap, make a nice smoothie with your favorite fruits. To top off the day, order in from your favorite restaurant. Go to bed early with a book or magazine and a bed tray of snacks or the leftovers!

48. Enjoy Your Food

The French have a saying derived from the lyric of an old French torch song: *Regret nothing in matters of love and food.* Puzzled scientists have been trying to figure out why the French have such low rates of heart disease in spite of a diet of heavy cream sauces (a situation known as the French paradox). They have found that the answer is passion. The French are passionate about their food and really enjoy it. They never think of food as sinful; instead, they simply think of it as tasty. To the French, food is a work of art, meant to be enjoyed.

To the North American, food means calories, fattening, and forbidden. North Americans tend to think about food as either fuel or poison; they fear the effect the food will have on their bodies. In France, good food feeds the *soul*, not just the body. In France, the idea of "food police" watching every gram of fat is mocked.

What the French also mock is the way in which North Americans eat: Everywhere and anywhere is a dining room. We eat in our cars, while walking on the street, and at our desks when we work. In France, eating takes place at restaurants or at dinner tables. The French consider the North American pattern of eating to be nomadic eating, or vagabond feeding and grazing.

There is also a huge distinction between quantity and quality of food. In North America, we are taught that large portions are good, even if the food is mediocre. In France, the quality and taste of the food are the most important factors. When the taste is excellent and the quality of the food is high, the appetite is satiated, and the quantity or portion size is not important.

When you enjoy your food, your body secretes endorphins, which relieve stress (see Item 32). One of the best-known comfort foods, chocolate, has demonstrated this effect.

49. Limit Your Exposure to Food Toxins

Enjoy your food, by all means. But environmental toxins place stress on our bodies, too. So if you can, try to have a safe food supply. Your weekly groceries probably contain residues from pesticides and other toxins, hormones in meat products, and a number of extras you may not have bargained for, but that were fed to your meat when it was still alive. These extras include feed additives, antibiotics, and tranquilizers. Meanwhile, most packaged foods contain dyes and flavors from a variety of chemical concoctions.

The quality of the environment also affects the quality of our food. Airborne contaminants, waste, and spills enter the water and soil, which, in turn, become part of virtually everything we ingest. In addition, when one species becomes unable to reproduce, the food chain is interrupted. Eventually, this comes to our kitchen tables. Cleaning up the food chain is all part of creating a healthy, contaminant-free diet for ourselves. So, before your next trip to the grocery, investigate the following questions:

- What did your food eat? Was it injected with anything? To find out, call the U.S. Department of Agriculture (USDA) information line: (202) 720-2791.

- What waters did the fish on your dinner plate swim in? The USDA information line should also have this information. For example, every time you eat fish that comes from one of the Great Lakes, you're being exposed to persistent toxic substances, particularly PCBs. The problem is that fish don't respect borders; so while Michigan fish advisories may ban one kind of toxic fish, an Ontario fish advisory may allow the sale of that same fish.

- Can you buy food that is organically grown? Look for a supply at local farmers' markets, natural-produce supermarkets, and in displays at your conventional supermarket.

- What was your produce sprayed with? To learn more about chemicals applied to conventionally grown fruits and vegetables, call the USDA information line.

- What are the produce-buying habits of your supermarket? You can find out by contacting your supermarket's head office.

Routes of Contamination

How do environmental contaminants get into our bodies? Here are the ways it can happen:

- *Food.* We know this because of tests done on feces, urine, saliva, breast milk, and other bodily secretions and excretions.

- *Drinking water.* We can check through bodily excretions and secretions.

- *Milk.* We can check through bodily excretions and secretions.

- *Skin (dermal exposure).* Absorption through the skin can be checked through sweat and hair samples.

- *Inhalation.* Inhaled contaminants can be measured with breath tests and all other bodily secretions.

Organic Growing

Organic growers are committed to ethical farming practices. According to many horticulturists and organic growers, the future of farming is called *sustainable farming*. This isn't anything new but, rather, centuries old! Sustainable farming creates a sustainable vegetation system or web that keeps rebuilding upon itself for decades to come. Planting in this way helps to renew and protect soil, allowing the diverse range of organisms—some even pests—to coexist within the food chain. When the food chain is left intact, parasites are taken care of by their natural predators or natural repellents.

Organic farmers therefore may practice *companion planting*, which is simply ethical biological pest management by arranging crops so that one type of crop can help another by protecting it from pests. Companion planting may confuse insects, repel them, or trap them. Companion planting is also used to make crops healthier. For example, one herb or vegetable may produce an odor that repels a beetle that is eating a certain crop, or it may be a more tempting treat for that beetle. Planting it near the crop provides protection, as well as possibly a second crop. Sometimes a farmer can even protect crops by allowing the growth of weeds with these beneficial properties. At the end of the season, the farmer harvests the crop and picks the weed, which can then be composted. In addition, certain vegetables, for reasons not completely understood, seem to thrive when grown near certain companion plants.

50. Cry More, Laugh More, and Learn to Forgive

Relieving stress comes from releasing stress hormones. One of the best ways to do this is through a good cry. Human tears contain high levels of stress hormone, which is one reason why people who cry tend to have less stress than those who do not cry. A dramatic movie can often induce tears, hence the term *tear jerker*, and this serves an important purpose.

Laughter is another way of releasing stress because it makes us feel good and boosts the level of endorphins, which combat stress hormones. Laughter also causes deep muscle relaxation (which is why you can sometimes lose bladder control). Blood pressure also drops, while the T cells in your immune system increase.

Incorporating humor into your life can be fun, too. Look for humorous books, magazines, or other materials, and keep them handy. Get yourself onto a humor listserv (unless it creates E-stress — see Item 6). Rent funny videos, watch comedy networks, and use laughter to diffuse stress at the office or at home. Laughter bonds people and also attracts people to you. Teachers, doctors, or salespeople who generate laughter have more loyal students, more compliant patients, and higher sales!

The final great stress reliever is forgiveness. When you have unresolved conflict with someone or you're nursing a grudge, the emotional weight you carry from the grudge when you think about the conflict increases blood pressure, stress hormones, heart rate, perspiration, and muscle tenseness. Forgiveness doesn't mean excusing bad behavior. Rather, it means that you are prepared to move forward and let go of your bitterness toward the other person. Forgiveness is healthier for you, and chances are, the person with whom you are engaged in conflict would either welcome your forgiveness or, if also nursing a grudge, would deep down want to forgive you, too.

Forgiveness is about saying the Serenity Prayer (accepting the things you cannot change, changing the things you can). You can't change the fact that the conflict occurred, but you can change your current response to that conflict. Here are some other things you cannot change:

- Other people
- Your age
- The way you were reared

- Death, illness, or an accident in the family
- Being laid off from a job

However, you can change some things:

- Your reaction to others
- Your goals
- Your self-esteem and self-worth
- The way you treat others
- The way you treat yourself
- Whether you communicate your needs to others

Epilogue

You now have in your hands 50 ways to reduce not only stress, but also your risk of virtually every illness. Since stress can predispose us to autoimmune diseases, cancers, heart disease and stroke, depression, and viral and bacterial infections, reducing stress can reduce all of that. By incorporating just one idea from this book into your life, you can reduce your stress levels. Whether by downshifting your lifestyle (Items 1 through 10), looking into hands-on healing (Items 11 through 20), applying what we know about nutrition and herbs (Items 21 through 30), making time for inner and outer workouts (Items 31 through 40), or taking care of yourself (Items 41 through 50), you can change your life for the better.

Bibliography

Allardice, Pamela. *Essential Oils: The Fragrant Art of Aromatherapy.* Vancouver: Raincoast Books, 1999.

"America's #1 Health Problem." *International Journal of Stress Management*, American Institute of Stress website, www.stress.org.

"Antidepressants' Impact Mainly from Boost of Getting Treated, Study Suggests." Associated Press, July 20, 1998.

Baker, Sandy. "The Number One Way to Eliminate Daily Stress." *National Public Account* 44 (Dec. 2000): 10–13.

Ballweg, Rachel. "7 Simple Ways to Reduce Stress." *Better Homes and Gardens* 78:62 (Jan. 2000).

Ben-Ari, Elia T. "Take Two Exercise Sessions and Call Me in the Morning." *BioScience* 50:96 (Jan. 2000).

——— . "Walking the Tightrope Between Work and Family." *BioScience* 50:5 (May 2000): 472.

Bennetts, Leslie. "E-Stress." *FamilyPC* 7:6 (June 2000): 93.

Bowen, Jon. "Fisticuffs in the Cube: Stressed-Out Office Workers Are Succumbing to 'Desk Rage.'" Posted on-line at www.salon.com (Sept. 7, 1999).

Bower, Peter J., et al. "Manual Therapy: Hands-On Healing." *Patient Care* 31, 20:69 (Dec. 15, 1997).

Carlson, Betty Clark. "Managing Time for Personal Effectiveness: Achieving Goals with Less Stress." *ISMA-USA Newsletter* 1 (Spring 1999).

Carlson, John G. "Relax Your Way to Stress Management." International Stress Management Association website, www.isma.org (June 2000).

Cass, Hyla. *St. John's Wort: Nature's Blues Buster.* New York: Avery Publishing Group, 1998.

Chaddock, Brenda. "Activity Is Key to Diabetes Health." *Canadian Pharmacy Journal* (Mar. 1997).

——— . "Foul Weather Fitness: The Hardest Part Is Getting Started." *Canadian Pharmacy Journal* (Mar. 1996).

——— . "The Magic of Exercise." *Canadian Pharmacy Journal* (Sept. 1995).

Christmas Derrick, Rachel. "Less Stress on the Job." *Essence* 30:11 (Mar. 2000): 44.

Cicala, Roger S. *The Heart Disease Sourcebook.* Chicago: Contemporary/McGraw-Hill, 1998.

Clarke, Bill. "Action Figures." *Diabetes Dialogue* 43:3 (Fall 1996).

Clarke, Robyn D. "Serenity Now." *Black Enterprise* 30:6 (Jan. 2000): 115.

"Combat Job Stress: Does Work Make You Sick?" Posted on-line at www.convoke.com/markjr/cjstress .html (Feb. 12, 1999).

Costin, Carolyn. *The Eating Disorder Sourcebook.* Chicago: Contemporary/McGraw-Hill, 1996.

Cotton, Paul. "Environmental Estrogenic Agents Area of Concern." *Journal of the American Medical Association* 271 (Feb. 9, 1994): 414–416.

Curtis, Patricia. "Stress-Free Zone." *Redbook* 194:6 (June 2000): 157.

Dadd, Debra Lynn. *The Nontoxic Home and Office.* Los Angeles: Jeremy P. Tarcher, 1992.

Datao, Robert. "The Law of Stress." International Stress Management Association, posted on-line at www.datodevelopment.com (June 2000).

Davis, Martha, Elizabeth Robbins Eshelman, and Mathhew McKay. *The Relaxation and Stress Reduction Workbook.* Oakland, CA: New Harbinger, 1995.

Delanet, Kathy, and Squillace, Marie R. *Living with Heart Disease.* Chicago: Contemporary/McGraw-Hill, 1998.

Douglas, Ann. *Sanity Savers: The Canadian Working Woman's Guide to (Almost) Having It All.* Toronto: McGraw-Hill Ryerson, 1999.

Dreher, Henry, and Alice D. Domar. *Healing Mind, Healthy Woman.* New York: Henry Holt and Co., 1996.

Engel, June V. "Beyond Vitamins: Phytochemicals to Help Fight Disease." *Health News* 14 (June 1996).

Evans, Julie A. "Stop Back Pain Instantly!" *Prevention* 151:7 (July 1999): 128.

Everyday Carcinogens: Stopping Cancer Before It Starts. Proceedings, Workshop on Primary Cancer Prevention, McMaster University, Hamilton, ON, Canada (Mar. 1999).

Farquhar, Andrew. "Exercising Essentials." *Diabetes Dialogue* 43:3 (Fall 1996): 6–8.

Ferraro, Cathleen. "New Uses of Chemicals Linked to More Illness." Scripps-McClatchy Western website (Dec. 10, 1997).

"A Field Guide to Stress: A Conversation with Kenneth R. Pelletier, Ph.D." *Selfcare Archives* (Dec. 15, 1997).

Franklin, Deborah. "The Return of Sunny Spring Isn't the Cure for All Cases of Seasonal Depression: Sometimes It's the Cause." *Health Magazine* website (1996).

Fransen, Jenny, and I. Jon Russell. *The Fibromyalgia Help Book.* St. Paul, MN: Smith House Press, 1996.

Fredman, Catherine. "How to Give a Back Rub." *Ladies Home Journal* 117:4 (Apr. 2000): 66.

Fugh-Berman, Adriane. *Alternative Medicine: What Works.* Tucson, AZ: Odonian Press, 1996.

"Get Herbal Relief." *Prevention* 51:7 (July 1999): 128.

Greenberg, Brigitte. "Stress Hormone Linked to High-Fat Snacking in Women." Associated Press (Apr. 4, 1998).

Grout, Pam. "Tune Out Stress." *Ingram's* 21:4 (Apr. 1995): 78.

Gunawant, Deepika, and Gopi Warrier. *Ayurveda: The Ancient Indian Healing Tradition.* Shafsbury, UK: Element, 1997.

Haas, Elson M. "Anti-Stress Nutritional Program." HealthWorld Online, www.healthy.net (June 2000).

Hendler, Saul Sheldon. *The Doctors' Vitamin and Mineral Encyclopedia.* New York: Fireside Books, 1990.

Herring, Jeff. "Bring Back Passion to Your Everyday Life." Knight Ridder/Tribune News Service (Feb. 21, 2000): 535.

——— . "Use These 10 Tips to Manage Stress." Knight Ridder/Tribune News Service (Jan. 31, 2000): 817.

——— . "You Can Manage Stress with HALTS." Knight-Ridder/Tribune News Service (May 22, 2000): 632.

Ho, Marian. "Learning Your ABCs, Part Two." *Diabetes Dialogue* 43:3 (Fall 1996).

Hoffman, David L. "Herbal Remedies and Stress Management." HealthWorld Online, www.healthy.net (June 2000).

——— . "The Nervous System and Herbal Remedies." HealthWorld Online, www.healthy.net (June 2000).

Hopson, Emma, and Judi Light Hopson. *Burnout to Balance: EMS Stress.* New York: Simon & Schuster/Brady Books, 2000.

Hopson, Emma, Ted Hagen, and Judi Light Hopson. "Emotional Support Can Help You Cope with Stress." Knight Ridder/Tribune News Service (Aug. 30, 1999): 7514.

"Hostility and Heart Risk." Reuters Health Summary (Apr. 22, 1997).

"How Forgiving Helps You." *Redbook* 194:3 (Mar. 2000): 36.

"How to Deal with Stress," posted online at www.back relief.com/stress.htm (Feb. 12, 1999).

Hunt, Paula. "Touch Up." *Vegetarian Times* (Nov. 1999): 96.

Iammetteo, Enzo. "The Alexander Technique: Improving the Balance." *Performing Arts and Entertainment in Canada* 30:3 (Fall 1996): 37.

International Food Information Council (IFIC). "Antibiotics in Animals: An Interview with Stephen Sundlof, D.V.M., Ph.D." Washington, DC: IFIC, 1997.

International Joint Commission (IJC). *Eighth Biennial Report on Great Lakes Water Quality, Under the Great Lakes Water Quality Agreement of 1978 to the Governments of the United States and Canada and the State and Provincial Governments of the Great Lakes Basin.* Washington, DC: IJC, 1996.

"Irritable Bowel Syndrome Linked to Emotional Abuse." *Tufts University Health & Nutrition Letter* 18:2 (Apr. 2000): 3.

Jahnke, Roger. "Breathing Practices." HealthWorld Online, www.healthy.net (2000).

———. "The Healer Within: The Four Essential Self-Care Methods for Creating Optimal Health." New York: HarperCollins, 1997.

———. "Qigong." HealthWorld Online, www.healthy.net (2000).

———. "Self Applied Massage." HealthWorld Online, www.healthy.net (2000).

Joffe, Russell, and Anthony Levitt. *Conquering Depression.* Hamilton, ON: Empowering Press, 1998.

Johnson, Catherine. *When to Say Good-bye to Your Therapist.* New York: Simon and Schuster, 1988.

Johnson, Lois Joy. "You Look Divine: Stress Management Techniques." *Ladies Home Journal* 117:92 (Jan. 2000).

Joplin, Janice. "The Therapeutic Benefits of Expressive Writing." *Academy of Management Executive* 114:2 (May 2000): 124.

Kaptchuk, Ted, and Micheal Croucher. *The Healing Arts: A Journal Through the Faces of Medicine.* London: British Broadcasting Corp., 1986.

Kaslof, Leslie J. "Natural Substances Offer New Hope for Stress Relief." HealthWorld Online, www .healthy.net (June 2000).

"Keeping Women in Line." *ABC News 20/20* (originally aired July 21, 1995).

Keyishian, Amy. "Calming Rituals for Rotten Days." *Cosmopolitan* 228:2 (Feb. 2000): 152.

"Kicking the Habit: At Last, a Treatment That Combats Craving." *Scientific American*, www.sciam.com (Jan. 2, 2000).

Kishi, Misa. "Impact of Pesticides on Health in Developing Countries: Research, Policy and Actions."

Paper presented at the World Conference on Breast Cancer, Kingston, ON (July 13–17, 1997).

Kock, Henry. "Restoring Natural Vegetation as Part of the Farm." *Gardening Without Chemicals* '91, Chapter 6. Toronto: Canadian Organic Growers (Apr. 1991).

Kotulak, Ronald. "Researchers: Lack of Sleep May Cause Aging, Stress, Flab." *Chicago Tribune* (Apr. 5, 1998).

Kuczmarski, R. J., K. M. Flegal, S. M. Campbell, and C. L. Johnson. "Increasing Prevalence of Overweight Among U.S. Adults: The National Health and Nutrition Examination Surveys, 1960 to 1991." *Journal of the American Medical Association* 272 (1994): 205–211.

Kushi, Mishio. *The Cancer Prevention Guide.* New York: St. Martin's Press, 1993.

Lad, Vasant. *Ayurveda: the Science of Self-Healing.* Santa Fe, NM: Lotus Press, 1984.

Lark, Susan, M. *Chronic Fatigue and Tiredness.* Los Altos, CA: Westchester Publishing Co., 1993.

Lemonick, Michael D. "Eat Your Heart Out." *Time* (July 19, 1999).

Lippert, Carol Gray. "Get a Life." Article A62599863, Financial Executives Institute (2000).

Liu, Lynda. "A Good Cry." *Teen Magazine* 44:6 (June 2000): 38.

Monhan Bartel, Margaret. "The Woods in Winter: Hiking as Stress Therapy." *Country Living* 7:2 (Feb. 1994): 65.

Mooy, Johanna M., Hendrik De Vries, Peter A. Grooten-
    huis, Lex M. Bouter, and Robert J. Heine. "Major
    Stressful Life Events in Relation to Prevalence of
    Undetected Type 2 Diabetes." *Diabetes Care* 23:3
    (Feb. 2000): 197.

Morrison, Judith H. *The Book of Ayurveda.* New York:
    Simon and Schuster, 1995.

Norment, Lynn. "Stress-Busting Secrets of Superbusy
    People." *Ebony* 55:9 (July 2000): 54.

Nyhout, Kristine. "Hands-On Relief." *Chatelaine* 73:6
    (June 2000): 45.

Ontario Task Force on the Primary Prevention of Cancer.
    Recommendations for the Primary Prevention of Cancer.
    Presented to the Ontario Ministry of Health (Mar.
    1995).

Pierpont, Margaret, and Diane Tegmeyer. *The Spa Life at
    Home.* Vancouver, BC: Whitecap Books, 1997.

Reing, Michael. "Stress and Genital Herpes Recurrences
    in Women." *Journal of the American Medical Association*
    283:11 (Mar. 15, 2000): 1,394.

Rifkin, Jeremy. "Playing God with the Genetic Code."
    Health Naturally (Apr./May 1995): 40–44.

Roberts, Francine M. *The Therapy Sourcebook.* Chicago:
    Contemporary/McGraw-Hill, 1998.

Roizen, Michael F., and Elizabeth Anne Stephenson.
    RealAge: Are You as Young as You Can Be? New York:
    Cliff Street Books, 1998.

Rosen, Larry, and Michelle M. Weil. *Technostress: Coping with Technology @Work @Home @Play.* New York: John Wiley & Sons, 1997.

Rosenthal, M. Sara. *The Gastrointestinal Sourcebook.* Chicago: Contemporary/McGraw-Hill, 1997.

——. *Managing Your Diabetes.* Toronto: Macmillan Canada, 1998.

——. *Women and Depression.* Chicago: Contemporary/McGraw-Hill, 2000.

——. *Women of the '60s Turning 50.* Toronto: Prentice-Hall Canada, 2000.

Rougher Arntz, Jane. "Under the Gun? How You Can Cope with Stress." *Business Journal-Milwaukee* 117:23 (Mar. 3, 2000): 18.

Seymour, Rhea. "Herpes Alert." *Chatelaine* 73:2 (Feb. 2000): 46.

Shimer, Porter. *Keeping Fitness Simple: 500 Tips for Fitting Exercise into Your Life.* Powal, VT: Storey Books, 1998.

Smereka, Corinne M. "Outwitting, Controlling Stress for a Healthier Lifestyle." *Healthcare Financial Management* 44:3 (Mar. 1990): 5.

Smith, Sand. "Pulling Your Own Strings: Three Keys to Personal Power." *OfficeSolutions* 17:3 (Mar. 2000): 44.

Sobel, David. *Mental Medicine Update* 4:3 (1995).

Spiker, Ted. "Choose to Snooze." *Men's Health* 115:4 (May 2000): 56.

"Stress Affects Your Health More than You Think." Posted on-line to www.mediconsult.com (Sept. 9, 1999).

"Stress-Busters: What Works." *Newsweek International* (June 28, 1999): 52.

"Stress May Intensify Cold Symptoms." Posted on-line to www.mediconsult.com (Mar. 26, 1999).

"Vacation of a Lifetime." *Time* 155:11 (Mar. 20, 2000): 92.

Vegetarian Resource Group (VRG). "Getting to the Roots of a Vegetarian Diet." Baltimore, MD: VRG, 1997.

Weed, Susun S. *Menopausal Years: The Wise Woman Way— Alternative Approaches for Women 30–90.* Woodstock, NY: Ash Tree Publishing, 1992.

———. *Wise Woman Ways: Menopausal Years.* Woodstock, NY: Ash Tree Publishing, 1992.

Weintraub, Amy. "The Natural Prozac." HealthWorld Online, www.healthy.net (2000).

"Writing About Stress Improves Your Health." *Research Digest*, posted on-line to www.mediconsult.com (June 16, 1999).

Zand, Janet. "Herbal Programs for Stress." HealthWorld Online, www.healthy.net (June 2000).

Zellerbach, Merla. *The Allergy Sourcebook.* Chicago: Contemporary/McGraw-Hill, 1995.

Resources

Body Work/Hands-On Healing

American Academy of Medical Acupuncture
   5820 Wilshire Blvd., Suite 500
   Los Angeles, CA 90036
   (800) 521-2262
   www.medicalacupuncture.org

American Academy of Osteopathy
   3500 DePauw Blvd., Suite 1080
   Indianapolis, IN 46268-1136
   (317) 879-1881

American Academy of Reflexology
   606 E. Magnolia Blvd., Suite B
   Burbank, CA 91501-2618
   (818) 841-7741

American Chiropractic Association
   1701 Clarendon Blvd.
   Arlington, VA 22209
   (703) 276-8800

American Massage Therapy Association
820 Davis St., Suite 100
Evanston, IL 60201-4444
(847) 864-0123, fax: (847) 864-1178
www.amtamassage.org; E-mail:
infor@inet.amtamassage.org

American Osteopathic Association
142 E. Ontario St.
Chicago, IL 60611
(800) 621-1773, (312) 280-5800
www.am-osteo-assn.org

Association for Network Chiropractic
444 N. Main St.
Longmont, CO 80501
(303) 678-8086

The Feldenkrais Guild
524 Ellsworth St., Box 489
Albany, OR 97321-0143
(800) 775-2118, (541) 926-0572
www.feldenkrais.com; E-mail: feldngld@peak.org

International Chiropractors Association
1110 N. Glebe Rd., Suite 1000
Arlington, VA 22201
(703) 528-5000
www.chiropractic.org; E-mail: chiro@erols.com

International Institute of Reflexology
Box 12462
St. Petersburg, FL 33733
(813) 343-4811
E-mail: ftreflex@concentric.net

Jin Shin Do Foundation for Bodymind Acupressure
1048G San Miguel Canyon Rd.
Watsonville, CA 95076
(408) 763-1551

Jin Shin Jyutsu, Inc.
8719 E. San Alberto Dr.
Scottsdale, AZ 85258
(602) 998-9331; fax: (602) 998-9335

National Center for Complementary and
Alternative Medicine
National Institutes of Health
8630 Fenton St., Suite 1130
Silver Spring, MD 20910
(888) 644-6226
nccam.nih.gov

National Certification Board of Therapeutic Massage
and Bodywork
8201 Greensboro Dr., Suite 300
McLean, VA 22102
(800) 296-0664, (703) 610-9015
fax: (703) 610-9005
www.nchtmb.com

The New Center College for Wholistic Health Education
& Research
6801 Jericho Turnpike
Syosset, NY 11791
(800) 922-7337, (516) 364-5533
fax: (516) 364-0989
www.newcenter.edu; E-mail: newcenter@d.com

North American Society of Teachers of the
   Alexander Technique
   3010 Hennepin Ave. S., Suite 10
   Minneapolis, MN 55408
   (800) 473-0620, (612) 824-5066

Nurse Healers — Professional Associates, Inc.
   175 Fifth Ave., Suite 2755
   New York, NY 10010
   (212) 886-3776

Office of Alternative Medicine Clearinghouse
   (for information about federally sponsored research
   in manual therapies)
   Box 8218
   Silver Spring, MD 20907-8218
   (888) 644-6226
   altmed.od.nih.gov

Rolf Institute of Structural Integration
   205 Canyon Blvd., Boulder, CO 80302
   (800) 530-8875
   www.rolf.org; E-mail: rolfinst@aol.com

Trager Institute
   21 Locust Ave.
   Mill Valley, CA 94941
   (415) 388-2688
   www.trager.com; E-mail: admin@trager.com

Counseling and Therapy Resources

American Association of Marriage and Family Therapy
    1133 15th St., N.W., Suite 300
    Washington, DC 20005-2710
    (202) 452-0109
    www.aamft.org

American Counseling Association
    5999 Stevenson Ave.
    Alexandria, VA 22304
    (703) 823-9800
    www.counseling.org

American Psychological Association
    Office of Public Affairs
    750 First St., N.E.
    Washington, DC 20002-4242
    (202) 336-5700
    www.apa.org

Center for Cognitive Therapy
    3600 Market St., 8th Floor
    Philadelphia, PA 19104-2649
    (215) 898-4100

Jonathan O. Cole Mental Health
    Consumer Resource Center
    McLean Hospital
    115 Mill St., Rehab. 113
    Belmont, MA 02178
    (617) 855-3298 or 2795; fax: (617) 855-3666

Justice in Mental Health Organization
United States of America
421 Seymour St.
Lansing, MI 48933
(517) 371-2266

National Institute of Mental Health
Public Inquiries
6001 Executive Blvd., Rm. 8184, MSC 9663
Bethesda, MD 20892-9663
(301) 443-4513; fax: (301) 443-4279
www.nimh.nig.gov; E-mail: nimhinfo@nih.gov

National Institute of Mental Health
Panic Disorder Division
Panic Disorder Education Program
Room 7C-02, Fishers Ln.
Rockville, MD 20857
(800) 64-PANIC

National Mental Health Association
1021 Prince St.
Alexandria, VA 22314-2971
(800) 969-6642, (703) 684-7722

Chronic Fatigue

Allergy Asthma Information Center & Hotline
P.O. Box 1766
Rochester, NY 14603
(800) 727-5400

American Academy of Allergy and Immunology
611 E. Wells St.
Milwaukee, WI 53202
(800) 822-2762

American Academy of Environmental Medicine
P.O. Box 16106
Denver, CO 80216
(303) 622-9755

American Chronic Pain Association
P.O. Box 850
Rocklin, CA 95677
(916) 632-0922

American College of Allergy and Immunology
800 E. Northwest Hwy., Suite 1080
Palatine, IL 60067-6516
(800) 842-7777

Candida Research Foundation
P.O. Drawer J-F
College Station, TX 77840

Center for Fatigue Sciences
28240 Agoura Rd., Suite 201
Agoura Hills, CA 91301

CFIDS Activation Network (CAN)
P.O. Box 345
Larchmont, NY 10538
(212) 627-5631

The CFIDS Association of America, Inc.
P.O. Box 220398
Charlotte, NC 28222-0398
(800) 442-3437 (44-CFIDS), (704) 362-2343
fax: (704) 365-9755
E-mail: info@cfids.org

CFS Crisis Center
   27 W. 20th St., Suite 703
   New York, NY 10011
   (212) 691-4800; fax: (212) 691-5113

Chemical Injury Information Network
   P.O. Box 301
   White Sulphur Springs, MT 59645-0301
   (406) 547-2255

The Cheney Clinic, P.A.
   10620 Park Rd.
   Charlotte, NC 28210
   (704) 542-7444

Chicago CFS Association
   818 Wenonah Ave.
   Oak Park, IL 60304
   (708) 524-9322

CompuServe CFIDS Support Area
   CFS/CFIDS/FMS Section (16)
   Health & Fitness Forum (GOODHEALTH)

The Connecticut CFIDS Association
   P.O. Box 9582
   Forestville, CT 06011
   (203) 582-3437 (582-CFIDS)

Fibromyalgia Network
   5700 Stockdale Hwy., Suite 100
   Bakersfield, CA 93309
   (805) 631-1950

National CFIDS Foundation
103 Aletha Rd.
Needham, MA 02492
(781) 449-3535, fax: (781) 449-8606 or
(781) 925-3393

National CFS & Fibromyalgia Association
P.O. Box 18426
Kansas City, MO 64133
(816) 313-2000

Sensitive to a Toxic Environment (STATE)
(for people with multiple chemical sensitivities)
The STATE Foundation
P.O. Box 834
Orchard Park, NY 14127
(716) 675-1164

Links

For more information about disease prevention and wellness, visit me on-line at www.sarahealth.com, where you will find over three hundred links, including the following emotional-health and heart-health links, related to your good health and wellness.

Emotional Health

International Society for Mental Health: www.ismh.org

National Institute of Mental Health (NIMH): www.nimh.nig.gov

American Counseling Association: www.counseling.org

American Association of Marriage and Family Therapy: www.amft.org

National Association of Social Workers (NASW): www.naswdc.org

American Psychological Association: www.apa.org

American Psychiatric Association: www.psych.org

National Center for Post Traumatic Stress Disorder (PTSD): www.dartmouth.edu/dms/ptsd/

The Anxiety Disorders Association of America: www.adaa.org

American Association of Suicidology: www.users.interport.net percent7Elindy/aas.htm

Canadian Mental Health Association: www.chmha.ca

National Alliance for the Mentally Ill (NAMI): www.nami.org

National Mental Health Association: www.healthtouch.com

Obsessive Compulsive Foundation: pages.prodigy.com/alwillen.ocf.html

Society for Light Treatment and Biological Rhythms (for SAD sufferers): www.websciences.org/sltbr/

Association of Gay and Lesbian Psychologists (AGLP): www.psy.uva.nl/

Mental Help (award-winning guide to mental health, psychology, and psychiatry on-line): www.mentalhelp.net

Depression Knowledge Center (put together by the World Federation for Mental Health, a comprehensive site offering FAQs, events listings, organizations list, archive, and discussion): www.depressionnet.org

AtHealth.com (mental-health links, chat, bulletin board, etc.): www.athealth.com

Mental Health Links (Web directory of useful links, associations, news and events, support, self-help, and managed care): www.mentalhealthlinks.com

CFS Days (for sufferers of chronic fatigue syndrome and fibromyalgia; offers information about signs and symptoms, research, diagnosis, treatment, and medications, as well as discussion and support group): www.sunflower.org/~cfsdays/cfsdays.htm

Mental Health at About.com (articles, forums, chat, and a newsletter, updated daily): www.mentalhealth.about.com

Online Dictionary of Mental Health: www.shef.as.ulc/~psyc/psychotherapy/index/

Walkers (information, a forum, and chat rooms for depressives and their loved ones): www.walkers.org

Chronic Fatigue Syndrome at About.com: chronicfatigue.about.com/health/chronicfatigue/mbody.htm

Internet Mental Health (information on disorders and treatment, with on-line diagnostic services and psychopharmacology index): www.mentalhealth.com

Mental Health Center (answers to many of the questions you may be too scared to ask): www.mentalhealthcenter.com

Heart Health

Heart and Stroke Foundation of Canada: www.hsf.ca

National Stroke Foundation: www.natstroke.asn.av

American Heart Association (official AHA site with heart and stroke guide, consumer information, and publications and news about all aspects of heart disease): www.americanheart.org

National Heart, Lung, and Blood Institute (NHLBI)
(publications and educational resources for
consumers and health care professionals):
www.nhlbi.gov/nhlbi/nhlbi.htm

The Beat Goes On (comprehensive site with chat and
information about drugs and treatment):
www.geocities.com/Heartland/Hills/2571/index.html

Becel Heart Health Information Bureau (the latest
information on nutrition, published for health care
professionals and the general public):
www.becelcanada.com

Adult Congenital Heart Association (information and
support resources for adults with congenital heart
disease): www.adultcongenitalheart.org

Arrythmogenic Right Ventricular Dysplasia (lots of
ARVD information, including articles, doctors' list,
and diagnostic products): www.arvd.com

Cardionet Program (cardiology education and
information program — highly specialized):
www.cardionet.hr

Global Cardiovascular Database (epidemiological
profiles of cardiovascular and cerebrovascular
disease in countries with emerging economies):
infobase.ic.gc.ca

Heart Listserve (E-mail chat group focused on heart
health): www.tinman.com/HeartList/cardchat.htm

Cholesterolbusters (natural ways to lower bad (LDL)
cholesterol and prevent heart disease, as well as
results of scientific surveys on cholesterol):
www.cholesterolbusters.com

American College of Cardiology (nonprofit medical society and teaching institution focusing on cardiac care and disease prevention): www.acc.org

Healthy Eating for Healthy Living (great information about how nutrition relates to heart disease): sln.fi.edu/biosci/healthy/diet.html

The Heart: An Online Exploration (interactive exploration of the workings of the heart, presented by the Franklin Institute Science Museum): www.fi.edu/biosci/

Cholesterol Site of the American Heart Association (information about managing your cholesterol, diet, and risks): www.americanheart.org/cholesterol

Just Move (American Heart Association's exercise site, with information, statistics, and self-assessment tools): www.justmove.org

Heartlink (charitable organization with on-line newsletter and lots of useful information, advice, and support): www.heartlink.org

One Among Millions (innovative site with useful information about prevention of heart disease): sln.fi.edu/biosci/healthy/disease.html

Women's Heart Institute (dedicated to prevention, evaluation, diagnosis, and treatment of heart and blood vessel disease in women): www.womensheartinstitute.com

The Cardiology Compass (navigation guide to cardiovascular information resources): www.cardiologycompass.com

Take Wellness to Heart (AHA women's website, offering women of all ages the facts on women's heart disease and stroke — risk factors, lifestyle issues, prevention): www.women.americanheart.org

Myheart.com (one-stop interactive resource designed to enable women to take charge of their heart health): www.myheart.com

High Blood Pressure (a complete guide, with clinically reviewed information, news, and discussion, plus good prevention tips): www.helioshealth.com

The Daily Apple Cardiovascular Center (expert health guide to all aspects of cardiovascular disease, including the latest news and information with emphasis on prevention): www.thedailyapple.com

HeartPoint (an in-depth look at cholesterol and how it affects the body): www.heartpoint.com/cholesterolmain.html

Doctor's Guide to Elevated Cholesterol (many articles, latest news, FAQs, discussion groups, and links): www.pslgroup.com/elevchol.htm

Index